50 LANDMARK PAPERS

every

Spine Surgeon Should Know

50 LANDMARK PAPERS

every

Spine Surgeon
Should Know

EDITORS

Alexander R. Vaccaro, MD, PhD, MBA

Richard H. Rothman Professor and Chairman
Department of Orthopaedic Surgery
Professor of Neurosurgery
Co-Director, Delaware Valley Spinal Cord Injury Center
Co-Chief of Spine Surgery
Sidney Kimmel Medical Center at Thomas Jefferson University
President, Rothman Institute
Philadelphia, PA, USA

Charles G. Fisher, MD, MHSc, FRCSC

Professor and Head, Division of Spine Surgery
University of British Columbia and Vancouver General Hospital
Director, Vancouver Spine Surgery Institute
Vancouver, British Columbia, Canada

Jefferson R. Wilson, MD, PhD, FRCSC

Neurosurgeon, St. Michael's Hospital
Assistant Professor, University of Toronto
Toronto, Ontario, Canada

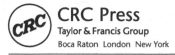

CRC Press
Taylor & Francis Group
Boca Raton London New York

CRC Press is an imprint of the
Taylor & Francis Group, an **informa** business

CRC Press
Taylor & Francis Group
6000 Broken Sound Parkway NW, Suite 300
Boca Raton, FL 33487-2742

First issued in paperback 2019

© 2019 by Taylor & Francis Group, LLC
CRC Press is an imprint of Taylor & Francis Group, an Informa business

No claim to original U.S. Government works

ISBN-13: 978-1-4987-6830-6 (pbk)

Visit the Taylor & Francis Web site at
http://www.taylorandfrancis.com

and the CRC Press Web site at
http://www.crcpress.com

Contents

Section One   Tumors

Section Two   Trauma

Section Three   Degenerative

Section Four   Deformity

Section Six   Pediatrics

Contributors

Reviewers

A. Karim Ahmed
Johns Hopkins School of Medicine
Baltimore, Maryland

Christopher S. Ahuja
Institute of Medical Science
University of Toronto
Toronto, Ontario, Canada

Tamir Ailon
University of British Columbia
Vancouver, British Columbia, Canada

Christopher P. Ames
University of California,
   San Francisco
San Francisco, California

Robert J. Ames
Shriners Hospitals for Children
Philadelphia, Pennsylvania

Howard S. An
Rush University Medical Center
Chicago, Illinois

Elsa Arocho-Quiñones
Medical College of Wisconsin
Milwaukee, Wisconsin

Ali Baaj
Weill Cornell Medicine
New York, New York

Jetan H. Badhiwala
University of Toronto
Toronto, Ontario, Canada

Sean Barry
Dalhousie University
Halifax, Nova Scotia, Canada

Michael R. Bond
University of British Columbia
Vancouver, British Columbia, Canada

David M. Brandman
Dalhousie University
Halifax, Nova Scotia, Canada

Joseph S. Butler
Mater Misericordiae University Hospital
Mater Private Hospital
Tallaght Hospital
Dublin, Ireland

Daniel Cataldo
Rothman Institute
Thomas Jefferson University
Philadelphia, Pennsylvania

Raphaële Charest-Morin
Laval University
Québec, Québec, Canada

Samuel H. Cheshier
Stanford University
Stanford, California

Simon Corriveau-Durand
Laval University
Québec, Québec, Canada

Chris Daly
Monash University
Melbourne, Australia

Nicolas Dea
Vancouver General Hospital
University of British Columbia
Vancouver, British Columbia, Canada

Peter B. Dirks
University of Toronto
Toronto, Ontario, Canada

Malcolm Dombrowski
University of Pittsburgh
Pittsburgh, Pennsylvania

Marcel F. Dvorak
Vancouver General Hospital and
    Vancouver Coastal Health
University of British Columbia
Vancouver, British Columbia, Canada

Richard G. Everson
David Geffen School of Medicine at
    UCLA
Los Angeles, California

H. Francis Farhadi
The Ohio State University Wexner
    Medical Center
Columbus, Ohio

Michael G. Fehlings
Toronto Western Hospital
University of Toronto
Toronto, Ontario, Canada

Charles G. Fisher
University of British Columbia and
    Vancouver General Hospital
Vancouver Spine Surgery Institute
Vancouver, British Columbia, Canada

Daryl R. Fourney
University of Saskatchewan
Saskatoon, Saskatchewan, Canada

Raj Gala
Yale School of Medicine
New Haven, Connecticut

Steven Garfin
University of California, San Diego
San Diego, California

Tony Goldschlager
Monash University
Melbourne, Australia

C. Rory Goodwin
Duke University Medical Center
Durham, North Carolina

Jonathan N. Grauer
Yale School of Medicine
New Haven, Connecticut

Akshay A. Gupte
University of Minnesota
Minneapolis, Minnesota

Raphael Guzman
Stanford University
Stanford, California

James Harrop
Thomas Jefferson University
Philadelphia, Pennsylvania

Roger Härtl
Weill Cornell Medicine
New York, New York

Gregory W. J. Hawryluk
University of Utah Hospitals and Clinics
Salt Lake City, Utah

Melvin D. Helgeson
Walter Reed National Military Medical
    Center
and
Uniformed Services University of the
    Health Sciences
Bethesda, Maryland

Sharon Husak
University of Saskatchewan
Saskatoon, Saskatchewan, Canada

Daniel S. Ikeda
The Ohio State University Wexner
  Medical Center
Columbus, Ohio

Christian Iorio-Morin
Université de Sherbrooke
Sherbrooke, Québec, Canada

W. Bradley Jacobs
Foothills Medical Centre
University of Calgary
Calgary, Alberta, Canada

Ajit Jada
Thomas Jefferson University
Philadelphia, Pennsylvania

Sukhvinder Kalsi-Ryan
Toronto Rehabilitation
  Institute–Lyndhurst Centre
Rehabilitation Engineering Laboratory
and
University of Toronto
Toronto, Ontario, Canada

Christopher Kepler
Rothman Institute
Thomas Jefferson University
Philadelphia, Pennsylvania

Erin N. Kiehna
University of Southern California
Los Angeles, California

Daniel R. Kramer
University of Southern California
Los Angeles, California

Tyler Kreitz
Sidney Kimmel Medical College
Thomas Jefferson University
Philadelphia, Pennsylvania

Jerry C. Ku
University of Toronto
Toronto, Ontario, Canada

Bornali Kundu
University of Utah Hospitals and Clinics
Salt Lake City, Utah

Mark Kurd
Sidney Kimmel Medical College
Thomas Jefferson University
Philadelphia, Pennsylvania

Shekar Kurpad
Medical College of Wisconsin
Milwaukee, Wisconsin

Joseph T. Labrum IV
Vanderbuilt University Medical Center
Nashville, Tennessee

James Lawrence
Albany Medical College
Albany, New York

Joon Lee
University of Pittsburgh
Pittsburgh, Pennsylvania

Stephen J. Lewis
Toronto Western Hospital
University of Toronto
Toronto, Ontario, Canada

Clifford Lin
Oregon Health and Science University
Portland, Oregon

Philip K. Louie
Rush University Medical Center
Chicago, Illinois

Jean-Marc Mac-Thiong
Université de Montréal
Montréal, Québec, Canada

Travis E. Marion
Vancouver General Hospital
University of British Columbia
Vancouver, British Columbia, Canada

Christopher M. Maulucci
Tulane University
New Orleans, Louisiana

Ryan P. McLynn
Yale School of Medicine
New Haven, Connecticut

Daniel Mendelsohn
Lions Gate Hospital
North Vancouver, British Columbia, Canada

Addisu Mesfin
University of Rochester School of
    Medicine and Dentistry
Rochester, New York

Andrew H. Milby
University of Pennsylvania
Philadelphia, Pennsylvania

Joseph A. Osorio
University of California,
    San Francisco
San Francisco, California

Markian A. Pahuta
Toronto Western Hospital
University of Toronto
Toronto, Ontario, Canada

Ann M. Parr
University of Minnesota
Minneapolis, Minnesota

Arjun V. Pendharkar
Stanford University
Stanford, California

Sina Pourtaheri
University of California, San Diego
San Diego, California

Kris Radcliff
Rothman Institute
Thomas Jefferson University
Philadelphia, Pennsylvania

Laurence D. Rhines
The University of Texas MD Anderson
    Cancer Center
Houston, Texas

Jonathan W. Riffle
Tulane University
New Orleans, Louisiana

Jeffrey A. Rihn
Rothman Institute
Thomas Jefferson University
Philadelphia, Pennsylvania

Theresa Clark Rihn
Sidney Kimmel Medical College
Philadelphia, Pennsylvania

Bryan Rynearson
University of Pittsburgh
Pittsburgh, Pennsylvania

Ahmed Saleh
Maimonides Medical Center
Brooklyn, New York

Amer F. Samdani
Shriners Hospitals for Children
Philadelphia, Pennsylvania

Carlo Santaguida
Montréal Neurological Institute and
    Hospital
McGill University
Montréal, Québec, Canada

Alexander Satin
Long Island Jewish Medical Center
New Hyde Park, New York

Rowan Schouten
Christchurch Hospital
Christchurch, New Zealand

Daniel M. Sciubba
Johns Hopkins University
Baltimore, Maryland

Andrew B. Shaw
The Ohio State University Wexner
  Medical Center
Columbus, Ohio

Jeff Silber
Long Island Jewish Medical Center
New Hyde Park, New York

Harvey E. Smith
University of Pennsylvania
Philadelphia, Pennsylvania

Hesham Soliman
Medical College of Wisconsin
Milwaukee, Wisconsin

Theodore J. Steelman
Walter Reed National Military Medical
  Center
and
Uniformed Services University of the
  Health Sciences
Bethesda, Maryland

James Stenson
Rowan University School of Osteopathic
  Medicine
Stratford, New Jersey

Godefroy Hardy St-Pierre
Hôpital de Chicoutimi
and
Université de Sherbrooke
Sherbrooke, Québec, Canada

John T. Street
Vancouver General Hospital
University of British Columbia
Vancouver, British Columbia, Canada

Geoffrey Stricsek
Thomas Jefferson University
Philadelphia, Pennsylvania

Daniel J. Sucato
Texas Scottish Rite Hospital
University of Texas at Southwestern
  Medical Center
Dallas, Texas

Ken Thomas
Cumming School of Medicine
University of Calgary
Calgary, Alberta, Canada

Alexander R. Vaccaro
Rothman Institute and Sidney Kimmel
  Medical Center
Thomas Jefferson University
Philadelphia, Pennsylvania

Peter G. Whang
Yale School of Medicine
New Haven, Connecticut

Andrew P. White
Beth Israel Deaconess Medical Center
Boston, Massachusetts

Jefferson R. Wilson
St. Michael's Hospital
University of Toronto
Toronto, Ontario, Canada

Alexander Winkler-Schwartz
Montréal Neurological Institute and
  Hospital
McGill University
Montréal, Québec, Canada

Michael M. H. Yang
Foothills Medical Centre
University of Calgary
Calgary, Alberta, Canada

Vinko Zlomislic
University of California, San Diego
San Diego, California

Introduction

For myriad reasons, there has been an exponential increase in the volume and quality of published research relating to spine care over the last several decades. Among thousands of articles, a small fraction has been shown to be truly *game changing*, forcing the entire field to pause and take notice. These landmark studies may describe a new procedure or surgical approach, evaluate the relative effects of known treatments or techniques, introduce a new classification system, or provide new insights into natural history or disease prognosis. While a number of these studies now are of historical significance only, they combine with more recent studies to form the foundations of spine surgery today.

The demands of a busy clinical practice or residency make it challenging to keep up to date with the burgeoning body of literature; therefore, our goal was to identify and summarize, in a user-friendly format, 50 of the most important studies in spine care. We anticipate that this book will be a useful reference not only to the established spine surgeon, but also to neurosurgery and orthopedic residents, as well as to spine surgery fellows as they continue to fortify their knowledge surrounding spinal disorders. Further, this will no doubt serve as useful evidence-based resource for trainees studying for professional examinations and perhaps most importantly challenge and inspire clinicians to produce high-quality impactful research.

The selection of studies to be included in the book followed a strict and multifaceted methodology. The first phase utilized bibliometrics to identify both citation classics (>400 citations) and emerging classics (>35 citations/year). The next phase involved the use of epidemiologic and methodological principles along with relevance and a comprehensive knowledge of the literature to refine the list of selected studies. Finally, 6 key opinion leaders who were named as section editors provided additional content expertise to finalize the 50 studies selected. Each of the section editors is recognized as a leader in their field of subspecialization. A complete description of methodology surrounding the study selection is described below.

Certainly, there will not be unanimous agreement or support from both the academic and nonacademic spinal community, of the 50 studies selected. Discussion and debate however can be a healthy and productive process. We also recognize that as time passes, and the volume of evidence expands, our list of landmark studies may require revision; that said, by including studies of high quality and enduring significance, we anticipate that this book will remain useful for many years to come. We sincerely hope that you derive as much pleasure in reading it, as we did in bringing it through to completion.

Methodology

1. A web-based search using Google Scholar and Web of Science was completed using search terms *spine, spinal, spine or spinal surgery, spine or spinal trauma, spine or spinal fractures, spinal cord injury, spine or spinal tumors, spine or spinal metastases, spine or spinal radiation, spondylolisthesis, scoliosis,* and *spine or spinal deformity.* Using the results from the described literature search we identified:
    a. Citation classics (those with >400 citations)
    b. Emerging citations classics (those with > an average of 35 citations/year)
2. A list of 100 *important* articles was produced based on a combination of: (a) the results of the literature search described above; (b) review of reference lists and bibliographies of articles identified in the literature search; and (c) discussion among the editors about articles of importance that were not identified through the literature search. The decision was made that articles of purely historical interest, with little relevance to modern spine surgery would not be included.
3. The list of 100 *important* articles was then distilled by the editors into a list of 50 *essential* articles with which every spine surgeon should be familiar. For organizational purposes, articles were classified under six main headings as relevant to:
    *   Tumor
    *   Trauma
    *   Degenerative
    *   Deformity
    *   Surgical Approach/Technique
    *   Pediatrics
4. Six section editors, identified to be content experts within one of the six main heading topics, were chosen to review the studies selected. The list of studies for each section was revised based on the feedback from these section editors.

Section Editors

1. *Tumor*: Laurence D. Rhines, The University of Texas MD Anderson Cancer Center
2. *Trauma*: Marcel F. Dvorak, University of British Columbia
3. *Degenerative*: Ali Baaj, Weill Cornell Medicine
4. *Deformity*: Christopher P. Ames, University of California, San Francisco
5. *Surgical Technique/Approach*: Steven Garfin, University of California, San Diego
6. *Pediatrics*: Daniel J. Sucato, Texas Scottish Rite Hospital

Direct Decompressive Surgical Resection in the Treatment of Spinal Cord Compression Caused by Metastatic Cancer: A Randomized Trial

Patchell RA, Tibbs PA, Regine WF, Payne R, Saris S, Kryscio RJ, Mohiuddin M, Young B. Lancet 366(9486):643–648, 2005

Reviewed by Christopher Kepler and Daniel Cataldo

Research Question/Objective   Prior to this study, radiotherapy and corticosteroids were recognized as the standard of care for the treatment of spinal cord compression caused by metastatic cancer.[1,2] In order to reevaluate treatment, the goal of this multicentered randomized trial was to assess the efficacy of direct compressive surgery plus postoperative radiotherapy versus radiotherapy alone for the treatment of spinal cord compression caused by metastatic cancer.

Study Design   This study was a randomized, multi-institutional, nonblinded trial where patients with spinal cord compression secondary to metastatic cancer were randomly assigned into either surgery followed by radiotherapy or radiotherapy alone. Before randomization, patients were stratified according to institution, tumor type, ambulatory status, and relative stability of the spine. Randomization within these stratified groups was performed at each institution with a computerized technique. The primary endpoint of the study was the ability to ambulate after treatment. Ambulation was designated as being able to take at least two steps with each foot with or without assisted devices. Secondary endpoints were urinary continence, changes in functional status utilizing the Frankel function scale score,[3] American Spinal Injury Association motor scores,[4] the use of corticosteroids and opioid analgesics, and survival times.

Sample Size   One hundred and twenty-three patients were assessed between 1992 and 2002 for eligibility. One hundred and one of those patients fit the criteria and were assigned into either group. Fifty patients were randomized into the surgery plus radiotherapy group, and 51 were randomized into the radiotherapy alone group. The patients were from 7 different institutions, including 70 patients from the University of Kentucky; 14 patients from MD

Anderson; 12 patients from Brown University; 2 patients from the University of Alabama–Birmingham; and 1 patient each from the University of Pittsburgh, the University of Michigan, and the University of South Florida.

Follow-Up   The median follow-up times were 102 days in the surgery plus radiotherapy group and 93 days for the radiotherapy alone group ($p = 0.10$). No patients were lost to follow-up in either group. Patients in both groups had neurologic assessments before surgery, weekly during radiotherapy, and within 1 day of the completion of radiotherapy. Patients also had additional regular study follow-up every 4 weeks until the end of the trial or death. This study was discontinued early because of proven superiority of surgical treatment. When comparing ambulatory rates between the two groups after treatment, the p value of 0.001 was below the predetermined significance level for early termination of $p < 0.0054$.

Inclusion/Exclusion Criteria   Patients must have been at least 18 years old with a tissue-proven diagnosis of cancer, which was not of central nervous system or spinal column origin. Patients must also have had MRI evidence of metastatic epidural spinal cord compression defined as true displacement of the spinal cord by an epidural mass from its normal position in the spinal canal. Patients had to have had at least one neurological sign or symptom, which could include pain, and not have been completely paraplegic for greater than 48 hours before entering the study. Additionally, the spinal cord compression had to be isolated to one area, which could include multiple contiguous spinal levels. Excluded from the study were patients with certain radiosensitive tumors such as lymphoma, leukemia, multiple myeloma, and germ cell tumors. Also excluded from the study were patients with preexisting neurological problems not related directly to their metastatic spinal cord compression and those patients who had recurrent metastatic spinal cord compression. Patients who had previously received radiation and were thus unable to receive the study radiation dose were also excluded. Last, patients had to have had a medical status acceptable for surgery and have an expected survival of at least 3 months.

Intervention or Treatment Received   Both groups were given the same dexamethasone regime, which consisted of a 100 mg dose given immediately, followed by 24 mg doses every 6 hours until the start of radiotherapy or surgery. Regardless of the group, treatment in the form of radiotherapy or surgery and radiotherapy was started within 24 hours after randomization. The total dose of radiation was 30 Gy in ten fractions, which was given to both groups. Surgical stabilization procedures were performed if spinal instability was present. Surgical approach and technique were tailored to each patient and the location of the tumor within the spine.

Results   After the completion of treatment, the ambulatory rate for the surgical group was 84% (42/50) and 57% (29/51) in the radiation group with a p value of 0.001 and an odds ratio of 6.2 (95% CI 2.0–19.8). Additionally, patients within the surgical group were able to retain ambulation for a significantly longer time than the radiation group (median 122 days versus 13 days, $p = 0.003$). When assessing the subgroup of patients who could walk at the start of the study, 94% (32/34) in the surgery group versus 74% (26/35) ($p = 0.024$) in the radiation group were able to continue to walk after the treatment. Within this subgroup, patients also continued to walk after treatment for a longer time in the surgical group versus the radiation group (median 153 days versus 54 days [odds ratio 1.82, 95% CI 1.08–3.12, $p = 0.024$]). Sixteen patients in each group were unable to ambulate at the start of the trial. Within this group of patients, 62% (10/16) in the surgery group and 19% (3/16) ($p = 0.012$) in the radiation group regained the ability to ambulate after treatment. In addition, within this subgroup, the surgical group walked for a median 59 days compared to a median of 0 days ($p = 0.04$) in the radiation group. Furthermore, surgical treatment versus radiation alone resulted in improved outcomes in urinary continence, ASIA motor scores, functional Frankel scores, mortality rates, corticosteroid and opioid analgesics, and length of hospital stay. The surgical group was able to maintain urinary continence for 156 days compared to the radiation group, for 17 days ($p = 0.016$). At 30 days, surgery group patients maintained or improved their pretreatment ASIA motor scores at a significantly ($p = 0.0064$) higher rate than the radiation group patients (86% versus 60%). In addition, at 30 days, the percentage of patients at or above the pretreatment functional Frankel scores was significantly ($p = 0.0008$) higher in the surgical group (91%) versus the radiation group (61%). The 30-day mortality rates were 6% and 14% in the surgical versus the radiation group, respectively, with a p value of 0.32. In the surgical group, the median mean daily dexamethasone equivalent dose was 1.6 versus 4.2 ($p = 0.0093$) in the radiation group. Additionally, the median mean morphine equivalent dose was 0.4 mg in the surgical group compared to 4.8 mg ($p = 0.002$) in the radiation group. Last, the median length of stay for both groups was no different (10 days) ($p = 0.86$).

Limitations   A possible limitation to this trial was patient selection bias. As with any study with extensive exclusion criteria, the results should be applied only to patients who meet the specific criteria outlined in this paper. An additional limitation is seen within the surgical technique because there were no standardized operative technique or fixation devices within the study.

Relevant Studies   Before radiotherapy was available, surgical treatment for spinal cord compression secondary to metastatic cancer was the treatment mainstay. With the advent of radiation therapy, several retrospective studies[5–10] and a small, randomized trial[11] demonstrated that laminectomy plus radiation did not seem to differ from radiation treatment alone. For this reason, surgical treatment was essentially abandoned. However, these studies focused only on laminectomy as the surgical treatment, which may not always be the optimal treatment for all patients. A majority of spinal metastases, which cause spinal cord compression, are found in the vertebral body. Therefore, laminectomy, which involves the removal of posterior elements alone, does not remove the tumor and thus often may not result in immediate decompression. Additionally, the surgical procedure can result in destabilization of the spine because often only the posterior elements are intact and their removal would lead to instability. For these reasons, this study proposed to reassess surgical treatment and radiotherapy versus radiotherapy alone.

REFERENCES

1. Byrne TN. Spinal cord compression from epidural metastases. *N Engl J Med.* 1992; 327: 614–619.
2. Loblaw DA, Perry J, Chambers A, Laperriere NJ. Systematic review of the diagnosis and management of malignant extradural spinal cord compression. *J Clin Oncol.* 2005; 23: 2028–2037.
3. Frankel HL, Hancock DO, Hyslop G, et al. The value of postural reduction in the initial management of closed injuries to the spine with paraplegia and tetraplegia. *Paraplegia.* 1969; 7: 179–192.
4. American Spinal Injury Association. *Standards for Neurological Classification of Spinal Injury Patients.* Chicago, IL: American Spinal Injury Association; 1984.
5. Gilbert RW, Kim JH, Posner JB. Epidural spinal cord compression from metastatic tumor: Diagnosis and treatment. *Ann Neurol.* 1978; 3: 40–51.
6. Black P. Spinal metastases: Current status and recommended guidelines for management. *Neurosurgery.* 1979; 5: 726–746.
7. Greenberg HS, Kim JH, Posner JB. Epidural spinal cord compression from metastatic tumor: Diagnosis and treatment. *Ann Neurol.* 1980; 8: 361–366.
8. Rodriquez M, Dinapoli RP. Spinal cord compression with special reference to metastatic epidural tumors. *Mayo Clin Proc.* 1980; 55: 442–448.
9. Findley GFG. Adverse effects of the management of malignant spinal cord compression. *J Neurol Neurosurg Psych.* 1984; 47: 761–768.
10. Sorensen PS, Borgesen SE, Rohde K, et al. Metastatic epidural spinal cord compression: Results of treatment and survival. *Cancer.* 1990; 65: 1502–1508.
11. Young RF, Post EM, King GA. Treatment of spinal epidural metastases: Randomized prospective comparison of laminectomy and radiotherapy. *J Neurosurg.* 1980; 53: 741–748.

CHAPTER 2

A Novel Classification System for Spinal Instability in Neoplastic Disease: An Evidence-Based Approach and Expert Consensus from the Spine Oncology Study Group*

Fisher CG, DiPaola CP, Ryken TC, Bilsky MH, Kuklo TR, Harrop JS, Fehlings MG, Boriana S, Chou D, Schmidt MH, Polly W, Berven SH, Biagini R, Burch S, Dekutoski MB, Ganju A, Okuno SH, Patel SR, Rhines LD, Sciubba D, Shaffrey CI, Sunderesan N, Tomita K, Varga PP, Vialle LR, Vrionis FD, Yamada Y, Fourney DR. Spine 15(35):E1221–E1229, 2010

Reviewed by C. Rory Goodwin, A. Karim Ahmed, and Daniel M. Sciubba

Research Question/Objective Although the indications for surgical management of metastatic spinal disease are well understood (metastatic spinal cord compression [SCC], progressive neurological decline), the concept of tumor-related spinal instability was previously difficult to reliably evaluate among surgeons and nonsurgeons alike given the complexity of spinal column biomechanics.[1,2] Given the lack of established guidelines prior to 2010, spinal instability in the setting of neoplastic disease was limited to the individual patient's subjective clinical experience combined with the associated physician's interpretation. Such subjective evaluation may result in inconsistencies in recognizing instability and may prevent clear and consistent communication among the members of the multidisciplinary treatment team, leading possibly to inappropriate or missed referrals for surgical management.[3]

As a result, the Spine Oncology Study Group (SOSG), an internationally recognized group of experts in spinal oncology, developed a classification system based

---

* Fisher CG, DiPaola CP, Ryken TC, Bilsky MH, Kuklo TR, Harrop JS, Fehlings MG, Boriana S, Chou D, Schmidt MH, Polly W, Berven SH, Biagini R, Burch S, Dekutoski MB, Ganju A, Okuno SH, Patel SR, Rhines LD, Sciubba D, Shaffrey CI, Sunderesan N, Tomita K, Varga PP, Vialle LR, Vrionis FD, Yamada Y, Fourney DR. A novel classification system for spinal instability in neoplastic disease: An evidence-based approach and expert consensus from the Spine Oncology Study Group. *Spine*. 2010; 15(35): E1221–E1229.

on review of available literature and expert consensus opinion to evaluate spine instability in patients diagnosed with neoplastic disease in 2010.[4]

Study Design   The SOSG first conducted two preliminary systematic reviews to identify clinical and radiographic factors associated with overt or impending instability involving tumors of the cervical and thoracolumbar spine. A modified Delphi technique was used to integrate the available evidence with expert opinion to develop the classification system. A questionnaire was then administered to the members of the SOSG that collected factors, based on individual clinical experience and review of evidence from the literature that contributed to spinal instability. A preliminary Spine Instability Neoplastic Score (SINS) was created based on the relative ranking of a particular factor's contribution to spinal instability. A second round of questionnaires involved more critical evaluation of instability factors, in an effort to improve reliability among evaluators and to improve validity of the score to predict instability in case examples. The SOSG ultimately defined tumor-related spinal instability as "loss of spinal integrity as a result of a neoplastic process that is associated with movement-related pain, symptomatic or progressive deformity, and/or neural compromise under physical loads."[4] Factors mentioned in the SINS included regional location of tumor, presence of mechanical/postural pain, bone lesion quality, spinal alignment, extent of vertebral body involvement/ collapse, and posterolateral involvement of the spinal elements.[4,5]

Sample Size   Not applicable. Three representative cases are presented in the text. However, the total series of clinical cases reviewed by the SOSG is not reported.

Follow-Up   Not applicable.

Inclusion/Exclusion Criteria   Not applicable.

Intervention or Treatment Received   Not applicable.

Results   The final SINS classification system includes six components, with a weighted value for each component. As such, the clinical presentation and imaging findings can be combined to determine an objective status of instability for a given patient with a neoplastic lesion of the spine. The score for each component is additive to achieve a final SINS. In terms of *location-specific factors*, junctional areas (occiput-C2, C7-T2, T11-L1, and L5-S1) are at the most risk for developing tumor-related spinal instability, with an assigned score of 3; the mobile spine (C3-C6, and L2-L4) is assigned a score of 2; the semirigid spine (T3-T10) is assigned a score of 1, and the rigid sacrum (S2-S5) is assigned a score of 0. With regard to *clinical pain presentation*, mechanical or postural pain is scored based on pain that may be relieved with recumbency (score of 3), while occasional, nonmechanical pain is assigned a score of 1, and a pain-free lesions score of 0. The *quality of the bone lesion* is scored based on whether the lesion is lytic (score of 2), mixed blastic and lytic (score of 1), or blastic (score of 0). *Deformity* is a major contributing factor and has the highest potential score, with subluxation/translation assigned a score of 4; *de novo* deformity, including kyphosis or scoliosis, assigned a score of 2; and normal spinal alignment assigned a score of 0. *Vertebral body collapse* is a score of 3 if it is greater than 50%, a score of 2 if it is less than 50%, a score of 1 if the lesion includes greater than 50% of the vertebral body but there is no collapse, and a score of 0 if none of the vertebral body criteria are met. *Posterolateral involvement of the spinal elements*, including facet, pedicle, and costovertebral involvement, may exacerbate spinal instability. If posterolateral involvement is present bilaterally in the neoplastic lesion, a score of 3 is assigned, unilateral involvement is given a score of 1, and involvement of the vertebral body without any posterolateral involvement is given a score of 0.

The maximum amount of points that can be earned is 18; a score of 0–6 denotes stability, a score of 7–12 is "indeterminate" and possible impending instability, and a score of 13–18 indicates instability. Surgical consultation is recommended for any patient with a score greater than, or equal to, 7.

Study Limitations   Although the study is currently the most comprehensive classification system for spinal instability in the setting of neoplastic disease, several limitations have been highlighted by the authors. Disease that is contiguous or multi-level, previous spine surgery, and previous radiation are relevant factors that can contribute to instability. However, these are not included in this classification system. Although the classification system is relatively straightforward, the study did not grade the representative clinical cases with spine surgeons outside the SOSG for reliability.[4] Although several additional studies have attempted to address these factors, most are retrospective in nature.[6–11] Prospective validation of this study will determine the SINS prognostic value in determining neoplastic spinal instability.[11]

Relevant Studies   Previous studies have attempted to quantify instability but have neglected to include key contributing factors or have only focused on instability using the framework created for spine trauma.[11–15] The Neurologic, Oncologic, Mechanical instability, Systemic disease (NOMS) and the Location of disease, Mechanical instability, Neurologic status, Oncological history, and Physical status (LMNOP) have incorporated the SINS criteria into the management paradigms of patients for patients with neoplastic spine lesions.[8,16] The interobserver and intraobserver reliability of the SINS classification system has also been widely demonstrated.[5,6,17,18] Furthermore, it has been determined to be more relevant for very radiosensitive tumors (i.e., multiple myeloma), where instability may be the primary indication for surgical intervention.[19] Additionally, a higher instability score has been demonstrated to increase the risk of radiotherapy failure for patients with metastatic spine lesions,[7] reinforcing the evidence for surgical stabilization among this high-scoring population.

Conclusion The SINS classification system is a useful tool to aid in determining neoplastic spinal instability. The original study provided reliable agreement and accurate evaluation of instability among members of the SOSG. Follow-up studies, done by multiple other author groups, now show this system may be valid among differing providers (e.g., radiologists, oncologists) and among differing clinical settings (e.g., histology-specific setting, following stereotactic radiation, etc.).

REFERENCES

1. Witham TF, Khavkin YA, Gallia GL, Wolinsky JP, Gokaslan ZL. Surgery insight: Current management of epidural spinal cord compression from metastatic spine disease. *Nat Clin Pract Neurol.* 2006; 2: 87–94; quiz 116.
2. Wood TJ, Racano A, Yeung H, Farrokhyar F, Ghert M, Deheshi BM. Surgical management of bone metastases: Quality of evidence and systematic review. *Ann Surg Oncol.* 2014; 21: 4081–4089.
3. Goodwin CR, Sciubba DM. Consensus building in metastatic spine disease. *Spine J.* 2016; 16: 600–601.
4. Fisher CG, DiPaola CP, Ryken TC, et al. A novel classification system for spinal instability in neoplastic disease: An evidence-based approach and expert consensus from the Spine Oncology Study Group. *Spine.* 2010; 15(35): E1221–E1229.
5. Fourney DR, Frangou EM, Ryken TC, et al. Spinal instability neoplastic score: An analysis of reliability and validity from the spine oncology study group. *J Clin Oncol.* 2011; 29: 3072–3077.
6. Fisher CG, Schouten R, Versteeg AL, et al. Reliability of the spinal instability neoplastic score (SINS) among radiation oncologists: An assessment of instability secondary to spinal metastases. *Radiat Oncol.* 2014; 9: 69.
7. Huisman M, van der Velden JM, van Vulpen M, et al. Spinal instability as defined by the spinal instability neoplastic score is associated with radiotherapy failure in metastatic spinal disease. *Spine J.* 2014; 14: 2835–2840.
8. Ivanishvili Z, Fourney DR. Incorporating the spine instability neoplastic score into a treatment strategy for spinal metastasis: LMNOP. *Global Spine J.* 2014; 4: 129–136.
9. Sahgal A, Atenafu EG, Chao S, et al. Vertebral compression fracture after spine stereotactic body radiotherapy: A multi-institutional analysis with a focus on radiation dose and the spinal instability neoplastic score. *J Clin Oncol.* 2013; 31: 3426–3431.
10. Versteeg AL, van der Velden JM, Verkooijen HM, et al. The effect of introducing the spinal instability neoplastic score in routine clinical practice for patients with spinal metastases. *Oncologist.* 2016; 21: 95–101.
11. Versteeg AL, Verlaan JJ, Sahgal A, et al. The spinal instability neoplastic score: Impact on oncologic decision-making. *Spine (Phila Pa 1976).* 2016; 41: S231–S237.
12. Asdourian PL, Mardjetko S, Rauschning W, Jonsson H Jr., Hammerberg KW, Dewald RL. An evaluation of spinal deformity in metastatic breast cancer. *J Spinal Disord.* 1990; 3: 119–134.

13. Denis F. Spinal instability as defined by the three-column spine concept in acute spinal trauma. *Clin Orthop Relat Res*. 1984; 189: 65–76.
14. Kostuik JP, Errico TJ, Gleason TF, Errico CC. Spinal stabilization of vertebral column tumors. *Spine (Phila Pa 1976)*. 1988; 13: 250–256.
15. Walker MP, Yaszemski MJ, Kim CW, Talac R, Currier BL. Metastatic disease of the spine: Evaluation and treatment. *Clin Orthop Relat Res*. 2003; 415: S165–S175.
16. Laufer I, Rubin DG, Lis E, et al. The NOMS framework: Approach to the treatment of spinal metastatic tumors. *Oncologist*. 2013; 18: 744–751.
17. Arana E, Kovacs FM, Royuela A, et al. Spine instability neoplastic score: Agreement across different medical and surgical specialties. *Spine J*. 2016; 16: 591–599.
18. Teixeira WG, Coutinho PR, Marchese LD, et al. Interobserver agreement for the spine instability neoplastic score varies according to the experience of the evaluator. *Clinics* (Sao Paulo, Brazil). 2013; 68: 213–218.
19. Zadnik PL, Goodwin CR, Karami KJ, et al. Outcomes following surgical intervention for impending and gross instability caused by multiple myeloma in the spinal column. *J Neurosurg Spine*. 2015; 22: 301–309.

CHAPTER 3

Spinal Metastases: Indications for and Results of Percutaneous Injection of Acrylic Surgical Cement*

Weill A, et al. Radiology 199(1):241–247, 1996

Reviewed by Alexander Winkler-Schwartz and Carlo Santaguida

Research Question/Objective   Metastases to the bone represent an increasing burden on health care resources worldwide.[1] Spine metastasis are particularly troublesome as they may contribute to a significant reduction in quality of life both from spine instability and pain.[2] Surgical intervention promises the potential of pain reduction as well as spinal stabilization. However, such procedures carry significant morbidity, especially when performed in a frail patient population burdened by extensive disease.[3] Percutaneous procedures obviate the need for high-risk surgery by providing a minimally invasive alternative to pain palliation and partial spine stabilization. Furthermore, they have the added potential of providing immediate relief of pain, compared to radiotherapy, which may take substantially longer to take effect. The goal of this study was to demonstrate the efficacy and risks of percutaneous injection of acrylic surgical cement in cases of spine metastases.

Study Design   Case series. It is presumed to have consecutively treated patients with prospectively collected data, but this is unclear.

Sample Size   Thirty-seven patients (20 men, 17 women, mean age 61.4 years) with spine metastasis underwent 40 vertebroplasty procedures. Eighteen patients were known to have single contiguous spine metastasis, with the remaining 19 patients having multiple sites of spine metastasis. Twenty nine of the 40 procedures were intended to treat pain alone and 6 of the 40 procedures were intended to stabilize the spine in addition to relieving pain. Five procedures were used solely to stabilize the spine (implying there was mild to no pain).

---

* Weill A, Chiras J, Simon JM, et al. Spinal metastases: Indications for and results of percutaneous injection of acrylic surgical cement. *Radiology*. 1996; 199(1): 241–247.

Follow-Up Until death of the patient or termination of study (mean 7.1 months). Six patients were lost to follow-up at 1–3 months.

Inclusion/Exclusion Criteria Inclusion criteria were painful metastatic segments or lesions threatening spinal stability. The decision to include or treat a patient was determined by a multidisciplinary team. Patients presenting with vertebral body height of less than one third were considered to be technically challenging and excluded from the study. Additionally, patients demonstrating any coagulation disorder were excluded due to increased risk of bleeding. If the posterior wall of the involved vertebral body was not intact, it did not necessarily exclude the patient to vertebroplasty. The number of individuals screened for the study were not stated in the manuscript.

Intervention Percutaneous intravertebral acrylic cement injection with fluoroscopic guidance. Eleven patients underwent multiple levels of vertebroplasty, and 2 patients required multiple interventions spanning 2 months to 2 years apart. Five of the 40 vertebroplasty treatments were performed in conjunction with an instrumented spine procedure. Ten vertebroplasty procedures were followed by radiation, and 7 were preceded by radiation.

Results Outcomes were divided into three groups: clear, moderate, and no improvement. Clear improvement was defined as a 50% reduction compared to the pre-procedure analgesic dose or a shift from narcotic analgesic to non-narcotic analgesic. Moderate improvement was defined as a decrease in pain without substantial gain in autonomy or a decrease of less than 50% of the pre-procedure analgesic dose.

Clear improvement was seen in 23 cases, moderate improvement in 7, and no improvement in 2. In the clear improvement group, 20 cases successfully stopped analgesics entirely. In 26 of 33 procedures, improvement was seen in the first 24 hours. Two procedures were not able to be assessed due to illness and death, and 5 procedures were excluded because the procedure was not per-formed for analgesia.

At 3 months, only 14 patients (15 procedures) of the initial 37 were available for follow-up. Five of these patients demonstrated a recurrence of pain. All cases of recurrence were related to progression of metastatic disease in adjacent verte-bral segments or pachymeningitis secondary to metastasis. Seven patients (eight procedures) were available for follow-up at 1 year, with one patient demonstrat-ing recurrence of pain.

Of the 10 patients (11 procedures) that underwent vertebroplasty for stabiliza-tion, 5 patients received instrumentation, and no patients were noted to have new instability at various follow-ups.

Two patients died within 15 days of the procedure, both of which appear not to be directly related to the procedure. Destruction of the posterior wall was noted in 40% of procedures. Twenty instances of cement leakage were noted. Of these, 5 patients demonstrated symptomatic complications, three radicular pain, and two dysphagia (out of 8 cervical procedures). Symptom relief was achieved within 72 hours with intravenous steroid therapy in both cases of dysphagia and one radicular (sciatic) pain. One case of radiculopathy required surgical intervention for the leak, with removal of the epidural cement. One patient remained with persistent radicular sciatic pain. There was one case of leakage of cement into the vena cava, which remained asymptomatic.

Study Limitations   The many flaws of this study are fundamentally related to the case series study design, which is largely descriptive and does not include a comparison group. Many of the limitations that will be listed below are implied and included for thoroughness and are not intended to detract from the importance of this paper. The patient population is not clearly described nor is the decision making to offer treatment clearly outlined. The details relating to the length of the recruitment period and number of patients that were screened for the study were not included. No references were made to how the data was collected and if there was research ethics board (REB) approval. There is no clear schedule for follow-up. The inclusion of patients undergoing multiple procedures, patients without pain, patients with heterogenous adjunct treatments (i.e., pre-radiation, no radiation, post-radiation, or instrumentation) makes the study difficult to apply to a specific population of patients. There are no validated measures for pain relief, quality of life, or performance status. There are no references to the definitions of adverse events and how the adverse events were surveyed. The loss of over 62% of participants by 3 months makes reliable conclusions about long-term outcomes problematic. Finally, the authors discuss results interchangeably in terms of patients and individual procedures, making the interpretation of their results difficult to follow.

Relevant Studies   The current manuscript demonstrates a significant paradigm shift toward minimally invasive percutaneous treatments, known as vertebral augmentation procedures (VAPs), for pain secondary to vertebral body metastasis. VAP was further refined with the introduction of balloon kyphoplasty as a means of restoring vertebral body height. In a 22-site, randomized controlled trial (RCT) as part of the Cancer Patient Fracture Evaluation (CAFE), 65 patients underwent kyphoplasty compared to 52 nonsurgical controls for the management in painful cancerous vertebral body fractures. At 1 month follow-up, the kyphoplasty group demonstrated statistically and clinically significant improvements in Roland-Morris Disability Questionnaire; SF-36 physical and mental component summary scores; back pain numeric rating scale; and Karnofsky performance status score; as well as a reduction in analgesic use, fewer cases of bed rest, and use of walking aids and back bracing. Thirty eight patients (73% of controls) in the control group crossed over to kyphoplasty after the 1-month assessment. Continuous improvements were seen in the kyphoplasty group until study termination at 12 months.[4] Given these results, kyphoplasty has gained favor as the principle VAP, though vertebroplasty remains a reasonable treatment for pain relief.[5]

REFERENCES

1. Pockett RD, Castellano D, McEwan P, et al. The hospital burden of disease associated with bone metastases and skeletal-related events in patients with breast cancer, lung cancer, or prostate cancer in Spain. *Eur J Cancer Care* (Engl). 2010; 19(6): 755–760.
2. Mercadante S. Malignant bone pain: Pathophysiology and treatment. *Pain*. 1997; 69(1–2): 1–18.
3. Eastley N, Newey M, Ashford RU. Skeletal metastases—The role of the orthopaedic and spinal surgeon. *Surg Oncol*. 2012; 21(3): 216–222.
4. Berenson J, Pflugmacher R, Jarzem P, et al. Balloon kyphoplasty versus non-surgical fracture management for treatment of painful vertebral body compression fractures in patients with cancer: A multicentre, randomised controlled trial. *Lancet Oncol*. 2011; 12(3): 225–235.
5. Papanastassiou ID, Filis AK, Gerochristou MA, et al. Controversial issues in kyphoplasty and vertebroplasty in malignant vertebral fractures. *Cancer Control*. 2014; 21(2): 151–157.

CHAPTER 4

Spine Update. Primary Bone Tumors of the Spine: Terminology and Surgical Staging

Boriani S, Weinstein JN, Biagini R. Spine 22(9):1036–1044, 1997

Reviewed by James Lawrence

Research Question/Objective   The authors' objective in this article was to address the variability of the terminology and staging of bone tumors of the spine by applying terms accepted by oncologists as applicable for musculoskeletal tumors of the limbs. In doing so, the authors sought to standardize the terminology by precise definitions and therefore foster improved interobserver communication and agreement. The authors present the Weinstein, Boriani, Biagini (WBB) Surgical Staging System as the culmination of these efforts and an expansion of the existing classification system pioneered by Dr. William Enneking, and subject it to clinical evaluation. Finally, the authors describe surgical planning methods in light of the WBB to aid in surgical planning for the treatment of spinal neoplasms.

Study Design   A partial literature review and review of oncologic staging, and a cogent explanation of the staging of spinal neoplasms in the context of prior staging systems with particular adaptation to the unique qualities of the spine.

Sample Size   Not applicable.

Follow-Up   Not applicable.

Inclusion/Exclusion Criteria   Eligibility of prior oncologic staging systems was not articulated in the manuscript.

Intervention or Treatment Received   Not applicable.

Results   The design of the paper begins with a clarification of surgical terminology as it pertains to musculoskeletal neoplasms. The authors define the terms *curettage, en-bloc excision or resection*, and *radical resection* clearly and differentiate among them to particularly highlight intralesional versus extralesional procedures, and offer stark contrasts between them. Of particular relevance to the spine, the authors describe *palliation*, which would represent surgical procedures performed with a functional purpose (decompression of the neural elements, stabilization of the spine), as occurring with or without partial tumor removal as an intermediary procedure. The authors also clarify that commonly used surgical terminology in spinal surgery, such as *vertebrectomy* or *spondylectomy*, are not oncologic terms per se unless accompanied by clarification using the otherwise specified terms. The authors then describe the oncologic staging system (developed by Enneking) in detail.[1,2] Based on a thorough preoperative workup including radiography, scintigraphy, computed tomography (CT), and magnetic resonance imaging (MRI), the system focuses on the extent of the tumor, its particularities on imaging, and its relationship with surrounding tissue (Figure 4.1).

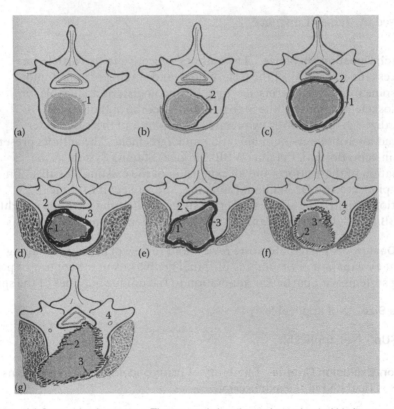

Figure 4.1   (a) Stage 1 benign tumors. The tumors is inactive and contained within its capsule (1). (b) Stage 2 benign tumors. The tumor is growing, and the capsule (1) is thin and bordered by pseudocapsule of reactive tissue (2). (c) Stage 3 benign tumors. The aggressiveness of these tumors is evident by the wide reaction of healthy tissue (2), and the capsule (1) is very thin and discontinued. (d) Stage IA malignant tumors. The capsule, if any, is very thin (1), and the psudocapsule (2) is wide and containing an island of tumor (3). (e) Stage IB malignant tumors. The capsule, if any, is very thin (1), and the pseudocapsule (2) is wide and containing of island of tumor (3). The tumoral mass is growing outside of tumor (3). The tumoral mass is growing outside the compartment of occurrence. (f) Stage IIA malignant tumors. The pseudocapsule (2) is infiltrated by tumor (3), and the island of tumor can be found far from the main tumoral mass (skip metastasis-4). (g) Stage IIB malignant tumors. The pseudocapsule (2) is infiltrated by tumor (3), which is growing outside the vertebra. An island of tumor can be found far from the main tumoral mass (skip metastasis-4).

The next section of the paper offers recommendations on safe and appropriate biopsy techniques. The authors suggest the transpedicular approach, as opposed to open surgical biopsy, which would otherwise contaminate other planes. The authors then offer a review of the existing oncologic staging system of benign and malignant neoplasms and their characteristics, also discussing the characteristic features of the natural history of the tumors of various oncologic stages, details of their appearance on imaging studies, and some aspects of their customary management. The section on benign neoplasms goes through the various stages (from S1 to S3), describing the increasing spectrum of aggressive behavior of these benign lesions, and the effects on surrounding tissue. Although expressed in generalities, the authors suggest typical surgical techniques to address these lesions and the use of adjuvant radiotherapy, cryotherapy, or embolization. For example, for S1 lesions, typically observation is performed unless *palliation* is needed for decompression or stabilization. S2 lesions are typically performed with intralesional curettage with or without adjuvant therapy. S3 lesions, which exhibit aggressive behavior including invasion of the surrounding compartments, can be treated with intralesional curettage with adjuvants (despite a high risk of recurrence), or marginal en bloc excision. Similarly, with regard to malignant neoplasms, the authors review the existing staging with regard to the lesions' inter- or extracompartmental status and the tumor grade. Lower-grade malignancies (Stage IA and IB) are treated with either an attempt at marginal resection with adjuvant therapy or wide en-bloc excision; higher-grade malignancies (Stage IIA and IIB) require wide resection and adjuvant therapy, although the authors note radical margins are not achievable in the spine due to the flowing tissue plane of the epidural space. Then authors then review their method of surgical staging to identify each lesion in a systematic fashion. This staging system vies each vertebra in the transverse (axial) plane and divides the vertebra in clock-face fashion (Figure 4.2). The longitudinal extent of the tumor is describing by numbering the involved segments. Classification of the tumor using this system again requires a synthesis of the relevant CT, MRI, and angiography (if performed)

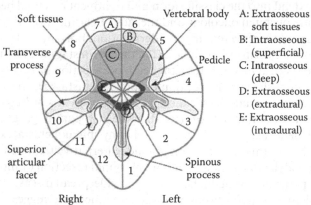

Figure 4.2 The Weinstein-Boriani-Biagini staging system. In this classification, the spine is axially divided into 12 equal segments and divided in 5 layers from superficial to deep. (Adapted from Boriani, S. et al., *Spine*, 22, 1036–1044, 1997.)

imaging. The authors highlight that the benefit of this system is that it accounts for the presence of the spinal cord in the longitudinal median axis of the spinal cord. The authors then highlight the three methods available for en bloc excision of tumors of the thoracolumbar spine: *vertebrectomy, sagittal resection*, and *resection of the posterior arch* in light of the staging system. Vertebrectomy is a procedure best performed for lesions largely confined to the vertebral body, in the parlance of this classification system, lesions confined to the 4–8 or 5–9 zones.

Study Limitations   The limitations of the study are essentially reflective of the time. In particular regard to the staging system itself, three-dimensional (3D) reconstruction imaging, such as we have today with computed tomography and 3D printing techniques, were not available to aid surgeons with this classification. Also of particular note are that the surgical methods seem particularly suited to the thoracolumbar spine and may not be easily extrapolated to the cervical spine, as the anatomy of the vertebral artery, the sympathetic chain, the thyroid and parathyroid glands, and the arterial anatomy further complicate the techniques of surgical resection. Newer surgical approaches, such as the *minimally invasive* transpsoas or oblique lateral approach, were not available at the time of the creation of this classification system. Larger and more morbid approaches, such as the open thoracic, abdominal, retroperitoneal, and transthoracic, may have a higher risk of tumor spread and certainly figure in the recommended approach for tumor resection, but were not options for surgeons at the time. Last, adjuvant care for spinal oncology has advanced significantly. The utilization of radiotherapy was limited by existing technology and greater morbidity but offers higher effectiveness for tumor care than was available at the time. In particular, sterotactic radiotherapy has emerged as both an adjuvant treatment as well as a primary treatment method for spinal metastases.[3]

Relevant Studies   Although Dr. Enneking's pioneering work in musculoskeletal pathology did extend into the classification and treatment of spinal neoplasms, the unique nature of spinal oncology and the lack of clarification of the terminology used at the time required modernization. Boriani et al., with this article, updated the classification and created their own staging system, which is used to guide surgical methods for either en bloc resection or palliative care. Tomita[4] in 2001 published a classification of spinal metastases in 2001 that accounts for the tumor grade, its location, and prognosis. According to this classification, patient evaluation was based on the histopathologic grade of the tumor, visceral metastasis to vital organs, and bony/spinal metastases. Points are awarded according to this classification to guide alternative treatment approaches from en bloc spondylectomy/wide resection, marginal resection or intralesional treatment. For patients scoring higher (i.e., with widespread disease or a poorer prognosis), palliative surgery, or observational treatment are suggested.

Tokuhashi[5] published a study in 2005 pertaining to preoperative prognostic classification for patients with spine metastases. The classification system was based on the patient's general medical condition, the presence of extraspinal bony metastases, the number of metastatic foci in the spine, and the patient's neurological status. Patients with a more favorable long-term prognosis are favored to undergo tumor resection, whereas more palliative measures are suggested for those patients with a poorer long-term prognosis. In 2010, the Spine Oncology Group presented the Spine Instability Neoplastic Score (SINS), a comprehensive classification system designed to create guidelines for referral of tumor patients to surgeons and to help foster improved communication among specialists with a particular focus on spinal stability in the presence of neoplasm.[6] Using an evidence-based design involving systematic reviews, expert opinion, and statistical analysis, the system uses the tumor location, the presence of mechanical or postural pain, the quality of the bone lesion, the spinal alignment, and vertebral body and posterior column involvement to create a composite score (Table 4.1).

Table 4.1 SINS

SINS Component	Score
Location	
Junctional (occiput-C2, C7-T2, T11-L1, L5-S1)	3
Mobile spine (C3-C6, L2-L4)	2
Semirgid (T3-T10)	1
Rigid (S2-S5)	0
Pain[a]	
Yes	3
Occasional pain but not mechanical	1
Pain-free lesion	0
Bone lesion	
Lytic	2
Mixed (lytic/blastic)	1
Blastic	0
Radiographic spinal alignment	
Subluxation/translation present	4
De novo deformity (kyphosis/scoliosis)	2
Normal alignment	0
Vertebral body collapse	
>50% collapse	3
<50% collapse	2
No collapse with >50% body involved	1
None of the above	0
Posterolateral involvement of spinal elements[b]	
Bilateral	3
Unilateral	1
None of the above	0

Source: Adapted from Fourney, D.R. et al., *J. Clin. Oncol.*, 29, 3072–3077, 2011.

Note: Data adapted.

[a] Pain improvement with recumbency and/or pain with movment/loading of spine.

[b] Facet, pedicle, or costovertebral joint fracture or replacement with tumor.

SINS: Spinal Instability Neoplastic Score.

SINS has proven to have excellent inter- and intraobserver reliability[7] and has become the standard for communication and classification of these lesions.

REFERENCES

1. Boriani S, Weinstein JN, Biagini R. Primary bone tumors of the spine: Terminology and surgical staging. *Spine.* 22(9): 1036–1044.
2. Enneking WF. Staging of musculo-skeletal neoplasms. In: Sundaresan N, Schmidek HH, Schiller AL, Rosenthal DI, eds. *Tumors of the Spine: Diagnostic and Clinical Management.* Philadelphia, PA: W.B. Saunders; 1990: 22–33.
3. Gucknberger M, Mantel F, Gerszten PC, et al. Safety and efficacy of stereotactic body radiotherapy as a primary treatment for vertebral metastases: A multi-institutional analysis. *Radiat Oncol.* 2014; 16(9): 226. doi: 10.1186/s13014-014-0226-2.
4. Tomita K, Kawahara N, Kobayashi T, Yoshida A, Murakami H, Akamaru T. Surgical strategy for spinal metastases. *Spine.* 2001; 26: 298–306.
5. Tokuhashi Y, Matsuzaki H, Oda H, Oshima M, Ryu J. A revised scoring system for preoperative evaluation of metastatic spine tumor prognosis. *Spine.* 2005; 30: 2186–2191.
6. Fisher CG, DiPaola CP, Ryken TC, et al. A novel classification for spinal instability in neoplastic disease: An evidence-based approach and expert consensus from the Spine Oncology Study Group. *Spine.* 2010; 35(22): E1221–E1229.
7. Fourney DR, Frangou EM, Ryken TC, et al. Spinal instability neoplastic score: An analysis of reliability and validity from the Spine Oncology Study Group. *J Clin Oncol.* 2011; 29(22): 3072–3077.

CHAPTER 5

A Revised Scoring System for the Preoperative Evaluation of Metastatic Spine Tumor Prognosis*

Tokuhashi Y, Matsuzaki H, Oda H, et al. Spine 30(19):2186–2191, 2005

Reviewed by Sharon Husak and Daryl R. Fourney

Research Question/Objective Metastatic disease of the spine is common and increasing in incidence due to improved detection methods and advances in the treatment of primary cancers.[1] While it is now widely acknowledged that decisions regarding the management of spinal metastasis must take into account many clinical, radiological, and patient factors, initial scoring systems developed to guide treatment of this condition were based on prognosis as the major determinant. The scoring system developed by Tokuhasi et al. for the preoperative evaluation of metastatic spine tumor prognosis is the best known of these systems and among the first attempts to predict the prognosis of patients with metastatic spine disease. The original scoring system was published in 1990 and based on six parameters: general condition, number of extraspinal bone metastases, number of metastases in the vertebral body, metastases to major internal organs, site of the primary cancer, and the severity of palsy.[2] The Tokuhashi score underwent revision in 2005 to assign greater weight to the primary cancer in the overall score. The goals of this study included evaluation of the accuracy of the total score in prediction, the relation of each parameter to prognosis, application of the score to conservatively managed patients (the original scoring system only evaluated surgically treated patients), and determination of any impact of lesion extension on the final score.

Study Design The authors describe the study design as being *semi-prospective* and, as such, the paper actually presents two separate analyses. The first is a prospective clinical study utilizing the revised scoring system, applied to data collected starting from 1998. The second is a retrospective analysis applying the revised Tokuhashi score to the

---

* Tokuhashi Y, Matsuzaki H, Oda H, et al. A revised scoring system for preoperative evaluation of metastatic spine tumor prognosis. *Spine*. 2005; 30(19): 2186–2191.

aforementioned prospectively collected data, as well as data previously analyzed under the original scoring system (collected from 1989 to 1998).

Sample Size   The total number of study participants in the prospective arm was 118, 36 of which underwent surgery and 82 of which received conservative (i.e., nonoperative) treatment. The retrospective analysis included a total of 246 patients (inclusive of the 118 participants noted above); 164 received surgery and 82 were treated conservatively.

Follow-Up   No mention of any standard follow-up schedule.

Inclusion/Exclusion Criteria   Patients with multiple myeloma and lymphoma were excluded. No inclusion criteria explicitly stated.

Intervention or Treatment Received   The revised Tokuhashi score is a sum of the points allocated for each of the six parameters evaluated (Table 5.1). The patient's general condition was assessed using Karnofsky's performance status (performance status of 80%–100% = 2 points; 50%–70% = 1 point; 10%–40% = 0 points). The number of extraspinal bone metastases was evaluated by both bone scintigraphy and MRI. In the case of a discrepancy between the two modalities, the greater number of metastases is used to calculate the revised Tokuhashi score (no metastases = 2 points; two metastases = 1 point; three or more metastases = 0 points). The number of vertebral body metastases was determined similarly (one metastases = 2 points; one to two metastases = 1 point; three or more metastases = 0 points). Chest CT, abdominal CT, and ultrasonography should be used to locate metastases to major internal organs whenever possible (no metastases = 2 points; removable metastases = 1 point; three or more metastases = 0 points), although the authors note that all of these tests were not possible in time-sensitive situations. The scoring for primary cancer was extended in the revised Tokuhashi score compared to the original to take into account its importance in predicting patient's survival periods (thyroid, breast, prostate, carcinoid tumor = 5 points; rectum = 4 points; kidney, uterus = 3 points; others = 2 points; liver, gallbladder, unidentified = 1 point; lung, osteosarcoma, stomach, bladder, esophagus, pancreas = 0 points). The severity of palsy was scored using Frankel's classification (Frankel E = 2 points; Frankel C, D = 1 point; Frankel A, B = 0 points).

According to the revised Tokuhashi score, patients with a score of 0–8, 9–11, and 12–15 have a predicted survival period of less than 6 months, 6 months or more, and 1 year or more, respectively. The revised Tokuhashi score, in combination with the opinion of the oncologist, was used to guide treatment. In general, patients with a predicted survival period of 6 months or less received conservative treatment. Patients with a predicted survival of 6 months or more underwent palliative surgical procedures (stabilization with or without

Table 5.1   Revised Tokuhashi Score

Characteristic	Score
General condition (performance status)	
Poor (PS 10%–40%)	0
Moderate (PS 50%–70%)	1
Good (PS 80%–100%)	2
No. of extraspinal bone metastases foci	
≥3	0
1–2	1
0	2
No. of metastases in the vertebral body	
≥3	0
2	1
1	2
Metastases to the major internal organs	
Unremovable	0
Removable	1
No metastases	2
Primary site of the cancer	
Lung, osteosarcoma, stomach, bladder, esophagus, pancreas	0
Liver, gallbladder, unidentified	1
Others	2
Kidney, uterus	3
Rectum	4
Thyroid, breast, prostate, carcinoid tumor	5
Palsy	
Complete (Frankel A, B)	0
Incomplete (Frankel C, D)	1
None (Frankel E)	2

Source: Adapted from Tokuhashi, Y. et al., *Spine*, 30, Table 2, 2186–2191, Copyright 2005.

Note: Criteria of predicted prognosis: Total Score (TS) 0–8 = >6 mo; TS 9–11 = ≤6 mo; TS 12–15 = ≤1 yr.

laminectomy), with the exception of patients with a score of 9–11 with only a single spinal lesion and no metastases to major organs, who were considered for excisional surgery (tumor excision with stabilization). Patients with a predicted prognosis of 1 year or greater underwent excisional surgery.

Results   The authors reported a survival period of less than 6 months in 89.0% of patients scoring 0–8, a survival period of 6 months or greater in 78.6% of patients scoring 9–11, and a survival period of greater than 1 year in 87.5% of patients scoring 12–15.

Study Limitations   One of the significant limitations of this paper is the study design and how it is presented to the reader. Careful reading is required to identify and separate the two analyses contained within. In addition, the actual analysis of the results is a bit muddied since the authors commonly combine a retrospective analysis of data initially evaluated in the 1990 paper with a retrospective analysis of prospective data, collected from 1998 onward. The data collected prior to 1998 was scored differently under the original scoring system, and the treatment associated with the original Tokuhashi score differed from the present study, which may confound the comparison of predicted to actual survival period. The only truly prospective data was the rate of consistency between the prognostic score and the actual length of survival for 118 patients; otherwise, the results derive from a combination of the two analyses.

Relevant Studies   Tokuhashi et al. published a subsequent article, further evaluating the revised Tokuhashi score in 2009, reporting the findings of a prospective study involving 183 participants.[3] This study evaluated clinical outcomes (improvement in pain and paralysis) and effect on activities of daily living (measured using the Barthel index) in addition to reevaluating the accuracy of the Tokuhashi total score in prediction of survival period. The authors reported a survival period of less than 6 months in 87.1% of patients scoring 0–8, a survival period of 6 months or greater in 87.2% of patients scoring 9–11, and a survival period of greater than 1 year in 95.0% of patients scoring 12–15. While these results were not statistically significant, the revised Tokuhashi score sparked much interest, and numerous studies evaluating its utility in predicting prognosis in patients with metastatic spinal disease have been completed.[4–7]

A variety of scoring systems to predict life expectancy for patients with metastatic spinal disease now exist, including the Tomita score,[8] the Bauer scoring system,[9] the Van der Linden scoring system,[10] and the Rades score.[11] These systems all include as parameters the site of primary cancer and presence of visceral metastases. Additional parameters are variable; however, there are some further commonalities between individual scoring systems. Unfortunately, none of these scoring systems are flexible enough to account for the effect of evolving systemic therapies and technological advancements (e.g., radiosurgery, kyphoplasty, minimally invasive surgery) on patient survival. Zoccali et al. reviewed the literature and determined that the accuracy of the revised Tokuhashi score has had a statistically significant decrease in accuracy over time for patients with an expected survival of less than 12 months, likely secondary to evolving treatments.[12] As an alternative to these rigid classification-based approaches, Paton et al.[13] published a principle-based decision framework called LMNOP that considers: (L) location of disease (anterior/posterior columns, spinal level); (M) mechanical instability as graded by the Spinal Instability Neoplastic Score; (N) neurology; (O) oncology (histopathologic diagnosis); and (P) patient fitness, patient wishes, prognosis (largely dependent on tumor type), and response to prior therapy. This systematic approach addresses clinical factors not directly addressed by other systems and is adaptable to changes in technology. Similarly, Laufer et al. proposed a neurologic, oncologic, mechanical, and systemic decisional framework (NOMS), adaptable to evolving technologies and systematic treatments.[14]

REFERENCES

1. American Cancer Society. Cancer facts and figures. American Cancer Society; 2007.
2. Tokuhashi Y, Matsuzaki H, Toriyama S, et al. Scoring system for the preoperative evaluation of metastatic spine tumor prognosis. *Spine*. 1990; 15: 1110–1113.
3. Tokuhashi Y, Ajiro Y, Umezawa N. Outcome of treatment for spinal metastases using scoring system for preoperative evaluation of prognosis. *Spine*. 2009; 34: 69–73.
4. Bollen MD, Wibmer C, Van der Linden Y, et al. Predictive value of six prognostic scoring systems for spinal bone metastases. *Spine*. 2016; 41: E155–E162.
5. Wibmer C, Leither A, Hofmann G, et al. Survival analysis of 254 patients after manifestation of spinal metastases. *Spine*. 2011; 36: 1977–1986.
6. Dardic M, Wibmer C, Berghold A, et al. Evaluation of prognostic scoring systems for spinal metastases in 196 patients treated during 2005–2010. *Eur Spine J*. 2025; 24: 2133–2141.
7. Wang M, Bunger CE, Li H, et al. Predictive value of Tokuhashi scoring systems in spinal metastases, focusing on various primary tumor groups. *Spine*. 2012; 37: 573–582.
8. Tomita K, Kawahara N, Kobayashi T, et al. Surgical strategy for spinal metastases. *Spine*. 2001; 26: 298–306.
9. Bauer HC, Wedin R. Survival after surgery for spinal and extremity metastases: Prognostication in 241 patients. *Acta Orthop Scand*. 1995; 66: 143–146.
10. Van der Linden YM, Dijkstra SP, Vonk EJ, et al. Prediction in survival of patients with metastases in the spinal column: Results based on a randomized trial of radiotherapy. *Cancer*. 2005; 103: 320–328.
11. Rades D, Dunst J, Schild SE. The first score predicting overall survival in patients with metastatic spinal cord compression. *Cancer*. 2008; 112: 157–161.
12. Zoccali C, Skoch J, Walter CM, et al. The Tokuhashi score: Effectiveness and pitfalls. *Eur Spine J*. 2016; 25: 673–678.
13. Paton GR, Frangou E, Fourney DR. Contemporary treatment strategy for spinal metastases: The "LMNOP" system. *Can J Neurol Sci*. 2011; 38: 396–403.
14. Laufer I, Rubin DG, Lis E, et al. The NOMS framework: Approach to the treatment of spinal metastatic tumors. *Oncologist*. 2013; 18: 744–751.

CHAPTER 6

Surgical Strategy for Spinal Metastases*

Tomita K, Kawahara N, Kobayashi T, Yoshida A, Murakami H, Akamaru T. Spine 26(3):298–306, 2001

Reviewed by Bryan Rynearson, Malcolm Dombrowski, and Joon Lee

Research Question/Objective   Surgical management for spinal metastasis is controversial. No clear consensus exists on deciding which patients should undergo surgery and what type of surgery is most appropriate. The primary goals of surgery are controlling the burden of local disease, preventing or slowing neurologic deterioration, and spinal stabilization when necessary. With the advent of more aggressive surgical procedures for spinal metastasis, the spine surgeon's armamentarium has changed. Preexisting scoring systems fail to account for these newer surgical procedures, and most do not guide appropriate treatment. As such, the authors proposed to develop a novel, comprehensive, prognosis-based scoring system to guide specific treatment in patients with metastatic spine disease.

Study Design   This study consisted of two distinct phases. Phase 1 represented a retrospective review of patients identified and treated for metastatic spine disease from 1987 to 1991. Primary and metastatic tumors were identified and evaluated via multiple imaging modalities including standard radiographs, bone scintigraphy, MRI, and CT scans. The region of the main spinal lesion was thoracic (39), lumbar (19), and cervical (9). The primary tumors were identified as cancer of the breast (14), kidney (12), lung (10), thyroid (9), colon (6), prostate (4), liver (4), stomach (3), uterus (3), and unknown (2). Three factors were utilized for a prognostic evaluation: (1) malignant grade of the primary tumor (as determined by tissue of origin), (2) visceral metastases to vital organs, and (3) bone metastases. Each factor was then subdivided to reflect varying degrees of clinical severity. Malignant grade of primary tumor (factor 1) was described as (1) slow growth, (2) moderate growth, or (3) rapid growth. Presence of visceral metastasis (factor 2) was described as (1) none, (2) present but treatable, or (3) present but untreatable. Bone

---

* Tomita K, Kawahara N, Kobayashi T, Yoshida A, Murakami H, Akamaru T. Surgical strategy for spinal metastases. *Spine*. 2001; 26(3): 298–306.

metastasis (factor 3) was described as (1) isolated to the spine or (2) not isolated to the spine. Finally, the relationship between length of survival and the aforementioned three prognostic factors was examined. Cox's regression model analysis and hazard ratios of each parameter were calculated.

Phase 2 represented a prospective study whereby a novel prognostic model utilizing the three factors described in phase 1 was used to determine appropriate treatment in patients who were treated for spinal metastases between 1993 and 1996. The primary tumors were cancer of the breast (16), lung (10), thyroid (8), kidney (8), colon (7), liver (3), stomach (3), prostate (2), uterus (2), and unknown (2). The region of the main spinal lesion was thoracic (34), lumbar (24), and cervical (3). Hazard ratios calculated for each factor group in phase 1 were rounded to the nearest integer and ascribed a relative point value in the scoring system. Using this strategy, a total score ranging from 2 to 10 was obtained for each patient. For a score of 2 or 3, wide or marginal excision was recommended, for a score of 4 or 5, intralesional excision ± marginal excision when possible was recommended. For a score of 6 or 7, palliative decompression and stabilization was recommended. Finally, for scores of 8 to 10, nonoperative palliative care was recommended. The treatment goal for each patient was set according to these numeric groups: long-term local control, middle-term local control, short-term palliation, and supportive care. Primary outcomes measured were type of intervention, length of survival, and local tumor control. The definition of local control was not explicitly stated but appeared related to recurrence of paresis.

Sample Size Phase 1 and phase 2 were comprised of 67 and 61 patients, respectively.

Follow-Up This was not explicitly stated in the article. However, the longest follow-up reported in either phase of the study was approximately 84 months.

Inclusion/Exclusion Criteria These criteria were not clearly stated in the article. However, the presence of metastatic disease involving the spine was present in all patients for both phases of the study.

Intervention or Treatment Received This information was only given for phase 2 participants and was as follows: 28 patients received wide or marginal excision (total en bloc spondylectomy (26), en bloc corpectomy (2); 13 received intralesional excision (piecemeal subtotal excision, eggshell curettage, or thorough debulking), and 11 patients received palliative decompression and stabilization. The remaining 9 patients received conservative palliative treatment.

Results

> *Phase 1*: The average survival period of 21 patients with a prognostic score of 2 or 3 points was 49.9 months (range 18–84 months); that of 13 patients with 4 or 5 points was 23.5 months (range 7–57 months);

that of 17 patients with 6 or 7 points was 15.0 months (range 5–33 months); and that of 17 patients with 8, 9, or 10 points was 5.9 months (range 1–14 months). Correlation coefficients between survival time and the three prognostic factors were calculated: grade of malignancy of the primary organs, -0.492 ($p < 0.0001$); visceral metastases to vital organs, -0.536 ($p < 0.0001$); and bone metastases, -0.250 ($p < 0.05$). The correlation coefficient between survival time and total prognostic score was the strongest at -0.690 ($p < 0.0001$).

Phase 2: The mean prognostic score for the wide or marginal excision group ($n = 28$) was 3.3 points (range 2–5 points), mean survival was 38.2 months (range 6–84 months) and 26 out of 28 achieved successful local control. The mean prognostic score for the intralesional excision group ($n = 13$) was 5.0 points (range 3–7 points), mean survival was 21.5 months (range 4–60 months), and 9 out of 13 achieved successful local control. The mean prognostic score for the palliative stabilization group ($n = 11$) was 7.5 points (range 5–10 points), mean survival was 10.1 months (range 3–23 months), and 8 out of 11 achieved successful local control.

Study Limitations   One significant limitation of this study is that it fails to incorporate patient comorbidities into the treatment algorithm. A comorbidity index, for example, the Charlson Comorbidity Index,[1] could prove a salient additional factor to further delineate treatment groups. Since inclusion and exclusion criteria were not stated in the study, it is unclear how patients deemed too sick for surgery owing to comorbid conditions were managed or if and how this treatment system can be applied in these patients. This may affect the applicability of this system; therefore, careful consideration must be taken on a patient-by-patient basis. Another notable limitation was that patient prognostic scores were not strictly adhered to with regard to the recommended surgical intervention. For example, 5 of the 11 patients that received decompression and stabilization surgery had scores of 8 or greater, for which this system recommends conservative palliative management. Numerous patient and surgeon-specific factors likely account for this discordance; however, the authors fail to acknowledge these discrepancies and how it could affect the interpretation of their results. Another important potential limitation is the failure to report the impact that radiotherapy and chemotherapy have on patient survival. It is not clear which patients had tumors sensitive to these adjunctive therapies and how many received these treatments in each of the four groups. The authors acknowledge the importance of these therapies on patient survival, but no discussion is offered explaining their rationale for excluding them from the scoring system.

Relevant Studies   The Tomita scoring system introduced in this study has become a popular clinical tool to guide therapy in patients with metastatic spinal disease; however, several other prognostic scoring systems have been described. These include, but are not limited to, the revised Tokuhashi,[2] Rades,[3] van der Linden,[4] Bauer,[5] and Katagiri[6] scoring systems. In contrast to the Tomita system, most of these systems aim to predict survival in patients only and do not have specific treatment recommendations. Other important differences among these systems exist as well. The Tokuhashi system, described in 1989 and revised in 2005, evaluates patient condition, number of spinal and extra spinal bony metastasis, operability of visceral metastasis, and neurologic status. It has been shown to be widely applicable, and its validity has been shown in multiple countries.[7] The Rades system, first described in 2008, has a narrower focus than the other systems and is applicable only in patients with advanced metastatic disease resulting in neurologic deficits that underwent radiotherapy. Its components are primary tumor type, presence of extraspinal bony metastasis, presence of visceral metastasis, interval time to spinal cord compression, ambulatory status, and timing of onset of neurologic deficits. The van der Linden system, described in 2005, is the simplest system and evaluates performance status, primary tumor type, and presence of visceral metastasis. The Katagiri system, also first described in 2005, is unique among these systems in that it incorporates prior chemotherapy use. However, it does not account for the extent of chemotherapy administration or the chemosensitivity of the cancer, which has resulted in problems with versatility and objectivity.[7] Finally, the Bauer system was first described in 1998 and includes primary cancer site, skeletal metastasis, visceral metastasis, and presence of spinal pathologic fracture. This system was revised to exclude pathologic fracture because this is often difficult to judge on imaging. The main drawback of this system is that it was derived from a multicenter cohort in which surgical indications varied widely, which could negatively affect its validity. Despite this fact, however, it has been shown to have good prognostic power in patients four or more years after treatment.[7]

Of these systems, the Tomita and Tokuhashi systems have the most abundant validity data, with several studies demonstrating their ability to predict patient survival accurately.[7-11]

REFERENCES

1. Charlson ME, Pompei P, Ales KL, MacKenzie CR. A new method of classifying prognostic comorbidity in longitudinal studies: development and validation. (0021-9681 [Print]).
2. Tokuhashi Y, Matsuzaki H, Oda H, Oshima M, Ryu J. A revised scoring system for preoperative evaluation of metastatic spine tumor prognosis. *Spine*. 2005; 30(19): 2186–2191.
3. Rades D, Dunst J, Schild SE. The first score predicting overall survival in patients with metastatic spinal cord compression. *Cancer*. 2008; 112(1): 157–161.
4. van der Linden YM, Dijkstra SP, Vonk EJ, Marijnen CA, Leer JW. Prediction of survival in patients with metastases in the spinal column: Results based on a randomized trial of radiotherapy. *Cancer*. 2005; 103(2): 320–328.

5. Bauer HC, Wedin R. Survival after surgery for spinal and extremity metastases: Prognostication in 241 patients. *Acta orthopaedica Scandinavica.* 1995; 66(2): 143–146.
6. Katagiri H, Takahashi M, Wakai K, Sugiura H, Kataoka T, Nakanishi K. Prognostic factors and a scoring system for patients with skeletal metastasis. *The Journal of Bone and Joint Surgery British Volume.* 2005; 87(5): 698–703.
7. Tokuhashi Y, Uei H, Oshima M, Ajiro Y. Scoring system for prediction of metastatic spine tumor prognosis. *World J Orthop.* 2014; 5(3): 262–271.
8. Kim J, Lee SH, Park SJ, et al. Analysis of the predictive role and new proposal for surgical strategies based on the modified Tomita and Tokuhashi scoring systems for spinal metastasis. *World J Surg Oncol.* 2014; 12: 245.
9. Liang TZ, Wan Y, Long GH, Zou XN, Peng XS, Zheng ZM. Predictive value of three surgical scoring systems for estimation of life expectancy in patients with extradural spinal metastasis. *Zhonghua zhong liu za zhi [Chin J Oncol].* 2010; 32(11): 875–879.
10. Zeng JC, Song YM, Liu H, et al. The predictive value of the Tokuhashi revised scoring system for the survival time of patients with spinal metastases. *Sichuan da xue xue bao Yi xue ban. J Sichuan University (Medical Science Edition).* 2007; 38(3): 488–491.
11. Aoude A, Amiot LP. A comparison of the modified Tokuhashi and Tomita scores in determining prognosis for patients afflicted with spinal metastasis. *Can J Surg [Journal canadien de chirurgie].* 2014; 57(3): 188–193.

Radiotherapy and Radiosurgery for Metastatic Spine Disease: What Are the Options, Indications, and Outcomes?*

Gerszten PC, Mendel E, Yamada Y. Spine 34:S78–S92, 2009

Reviewed by Simon Corriveau-Durand and Raphaële Charest-Morin

Research Question/Objective   The role of conventional radiotherapy (CRT) for metastatic tumors of the spine is well established. Over the last decade, stereotactic body radiosurgery (SBRS) has emerged as an alternative option, shifting the treatment paradigm in the management of spinal metastases. The objective of this publication was to provide an evidence-based overview of the best available literature on three clinically relevant questions related to the use of SBRS and CRT:

1. What are the clinical outcomes of the current indications?
2. What are the current dose recommendations and fractionation schedules?
3. What are the current known patterns of failure and complications?

Study Design   A systematic literature review on CRT and SBRS in the management of spinal metastases was undertaken using PubMed, Embase, and the Cochrane evidence-based medicine database. Articles in the English-language literature were reviewed, and references from each publication were searched for additional articles. Clinically relevant questions were elaborated by the Spine Oncology Study Group (SOSG), a multidisciplinary panel of experts and recommendations were issued using the GRADE methodology popularized by Guyatt et al.[1] Recommendations are either strong or weak and are based on the quality of the evidence and clinical expertise.

Sample Size   For CRT, 49 studies met the inclusion criteria; 3 randomized trials (high-quality of evidence), 4 prospective studies (moderate

---

* Gerszten PC, Mendel E, Yamada Y. Radiotherapy and radiosurgery for metastatic spine disease: What are the options, indications, and outcomes? *Spine.* 2009; 34: S78–S92.

quality of evidence) and 42 nonprospective studies (low or very low quality of evidence) with a total over 5000 patients.

For SBRS, 29 articles referring to spine radiosurgery for metastatic spine disease alone or in combination with benign spinal tumors were identified (low and very low quality of evidence). No randomized trials were available.

Follow-Up Not applicable.

Inclusion/Exclusion Criteria Inclusion criteria included articles relevant to CRT or SBRS in the treatment of metastatic spine disease. Data published before 1980, as well as publications describing less than 10 patients, were excluded. Articles elaborating primarily surgical treatment and/or without radiation therapy data were excluded. Surgical data describing cohorts who had radiotherapy without surgery were included if sufficient information regarding radiation and outcomes was provided.

Intervention or Treatment Received Patients included in this systematic review underwent either CRT or SBRS for metastatic spine disease. As no standardized treatment exists, there was a large heterogeneity of radiation regimen received by the patients.

Results
1. What are the clinical outcomes of the current indications?
   After CRT for epidural cord compression, 60%–80% of patients remained ambulatory. Ability for nonambulant patients to walk after radiation showed wide variation (20%–60%), and studies with higher level of evidence showed less optimistic results (19%–33%). With regard to pain, between 50% and 70% of the patients demonstrated improvement following CRT. However, no validated instruments were used, and length of follow-up varied significantly. SBRS has been reported as a highly effective modality to decrease pain in up to 85%–100% of patients. Durable pain improvement and maintained health-related quality of life (HRQOL) have been reported, even with radio-resistant histologies. In the setting of progressive neurologic deficit where surgery was contraindicated, 57%–92% of the patient experienced neurologic improvement following SBRS.
2. What are the current dose recommendations and fractionation schedules?
   For CRT, various regimens have been reported. Three prospective studies failed to demonstrate that dose fractionation schedule has an impact on ambulation. Retrospective data suggest that a longer course (>1 week) offers better motor function score compared to a shorter course (<1 week). However, a shorter course may still be indicated for patients with a limited life expectancy. For SBRS, all dose regimens appear to be safe and efficacious, and no recommendation of one regimen over another was made.

3. What are the current known patterns of failure and complications?
   Local control defined as the absence of recurrent cord compression was
   achieved in 61%–89%, with a mean of 77% for CRT. Tumor histology represents an important prognostic factor: lymphoma, seminoma, myeloma,
   breast cancer, and prostate cancer are favorable histologies, whereas sar-
   comas, melanomas, renal cell carcinomas, gastrointestinal carcinoma, and
   non-small cell lung cancer (NSCLC) are unfavorable. In term of toxicity,
   CRT appears to be safe, and one case of radiation myelopathy has been
   described. Excellent local control rate of approximately 90% has been
   reported (75%–100%) with SBRS. SBRS was used as a primary treatment, as
   a re-irradiation procedure, or as an adjuvant to surgery. Progression occurring at adjacent levels is rare, but progression at the epidural space has been
   described. Radiation myelopathy has been reported in seven cases.

SOSG Recommendations
1. CRT is indicated for the treatment of spinal metastases in the absence of
   instability, prior radiation, high-grade cord compression, and radio-resistant
   histology (strong recommendation, moderate-quality evidence).
2. SBRS should be considered over CRT in the setting of oligometastatic disease and/or radio-resistant histology when no relative contraindications exist
   (strong recommendation, low-quality evidence).

Study Limitations   The metastatic spine population is a difficult group
to study given its heterogeneity. Direct impact of a treatment is difficult
to distinguish over another one. Patient survival is also limited in this
population, and length of follow-up in the reported literature varies
widely. Different outcome measures were used and none is specific to the
metastatic spine population. Therefore, comparison between studies is
difficult. Few articles reported results with the SF-36 or ECOG, which
are valid and reliable instruments for the oncologic population.[2] Since
this publication, the SOSG has developed a specific HRQoL outcome
tool for the metastatic spine population that may enable the clinician to
better assess the well-being of that population.[3] Most of the publications
included in this article are retrospective studies with a methodological
quality qualified as *overall low*. However, most of their results are
consistent and in accordance with the higher level of evidence articles.

Relevant Studies   Recently, in 2015, a Cochrane Review was published on
metastatic extradural spinal cord compression in which was included seven
randomized controlled trials (RCT) (876 patients).[4] Their results showed
similar outcomes for CRT: ambulation status between 65% and 69%, reduction
of narcotic use between 34% and 40%, and maintenance of bowel and bladder
function between 87% and 80%. There was no significant difference between
radiation schedules (single dose, short course, and split course). Tumor recurrence

was slightly higher with single dose compared to split course or short course, but it didn't reach statistical significance. No serious adverse events were reported.

There is a growing body of literature supporting SBRS in the treatment of spinal metastases. This translates into clinical care with treatment shifting from surgery to SBRS. A good example is the solitary renal metastases; with local control rate with SBRS similar to en bloc resection (6%–13% versus 7.5%), Bilsky et al.[5] have been advocating for SRBS as a first line of treatment when there is no epidural compression and thus as a way of avoiding the morbidity of an en bloc resection.

With the advance of SBRS and its widespread use, it is now known that local control is significantly better when the epidural disease is low grade.[6] Using the Bilsky classification,[7] high-grade compression is defined by deformation of the spinal cord with or without persistence of visible cerebrospinal fluid. This has led to the development of separation surgery, where the epidural disease is downgraded surgically to enable effective and rapid postoperative SBRS. Good local control and an acceptable complication rate have been reported.[8,9] Vertebral compression fractures (VCFs) have been documented as a late complication following SBRS. An occurrence between 11% and 39% has been reported and risk factors identified: lytic lesion, malalignment, 20 Gy or greater per fraction.[10–12] Most of these fracture occurred within 4 months. Pre-SBRT cement augmentation could be considered in these patients to decrease the risk of subsequent VCF. However, nearly half of these fractures remain asymptomatic and therefore do not require treatment.[13]

REFERENCES

1. Schunemann HJ, Jaeschke R, Cook DJ, et al. An official ATS statement: Grading the quality of evidence and strength of recommendations in ATS guidelines and recommendations. *Am J Respir Crit Care Med.* 2006; 174: 605–614.
2. Street J, Berven S, Fisher C, Ryken T. Health-related quality of life assessment in metastatic disease of the spine: A systematic review. *Spine.* 2009; 34: 22S, S128–S134.
3. Street J, Lenehan B, Berven S, Fisher C. Introducing a new health-related quality of life outcome tool for metastatic disease of the spine: Content validation using the international classification of functioning, disability, and health; on behalf of the Spine Oncology Study Group. *Spine.* 2010; 35: 14, 1377–1386.
4. George R, Jeba J, Ramkumar G, Chacko AG, Tharyan P. Interventions for the treatment of metastatic extradural spinal cord compression in adults (Review). *The Cochrane Library.* 2015; 9.
5. Bilsky MH, Laufer I, Burch S. Shifting paradigms in the treatment of metastatic spine disease. *Spine.* 2009; 34: 22S, S101–S107.
6. Al-Omair A, Masucci L, Masson-Cote L, et al. Surgical resection of epidural disease improves local control following postoperative spine stereotactic body radiotherapy. *Neuro Oncol.* 2013; 15(10): 1413–1419.

7. Bilsky MH, Laufer I, Fourney DR, et al. Reliability analysis of the epidural spinal cord compression scale. *J Neurosurg Spine.* 2010; 13(3): 324–328.
8. Laufer I, Iorgulescu JB, Chapman T, et al. Local disease control for spinal metastases following "separation surgery" and adjuvant hypofractionated or high-dose single-fraction stereotactic radiosurgery: Outcome analysis in 186 patients. *J Neurosurg Spine.* 2013; 18(3): 207–214.
9. Bate BG, Khan NR, Kimball BY, Gabrick K, Weaver J. Stereotactic radiosurgery for spinal metastases with or without separation surgery. *J Neurosurg Spine.* 2015; 22(4): 409–415.
10. Sahgal A, Whyne CM, Ma L, Larson DA, Fehlings MG. Vertebral compression fracture after stereotactic body radiotherapy for spinal metastases. *Lancet Oncol.* 2013; 14: e310–e320.
11. Cunha MV, Al-Omair A, Atenafu EG, et al. Vertebral compression fracture (VCF) after spine stereotactic body radiation therapy (SBRT): Analysis of predictive factors. *Int J Radiat Oncol Biol Phys* 2012; 84: e343–e349.
12. Jawad MS, Fahim DK, Gerszten PC, et al. Vertebral compression fractures after stereotactic body radiation therapy: A large, multi-institutional, multinational evaluation. *J Neurosurg Spine.* 2016.
13. Sahgal A, Atenafu EG, Chao S, et al. Vertebral compression fracture after spine stereotactic body radiotherapy: A multi-institutional analysis with a focus on radiation dose and the spinal instability neoplastic score. *J Clin Oncol.* 2013; 31(27): 3426–3431.

Feasibility and Safety of En Bloc Resection for Primary Spine Tumors: A Systematic Review by the Spine Oncology Study Group*

Yamazaki T, McLoughlin GS, Patel S, Rhines LD, Fourney DR. Spine 34:S31–S38, 2009

Reviewed by Richard G. Everson and Laurence D. Rhines

Research Question/Objective   The application of surgical oncologic principles to the resection of primary malignant tumors of the spine requires consideration of en bloc resection—where a tumor is removed in a single, intact piece, fully encased by a continuous layer of normal tissue—to offer the best chance of disease-free survival. However, since surgeries performed with this technique are technically challenging, resource intensive, and associated with early morbidity, their adoption was met with reluctance in the spine community. Procedures performed in nonspecialty centers often resulted in contaminated margins, which were felt to cause higher rates of recurrence as well as complicate and reduce the effectiveness of more definitive resection. The purposes of this study were to determine the effect of incisional biopsy prior to resection, and to present the cumulative results of studies reporting en bloc resection in order to weigh the impact of achieving appropriate surgical margins against the perceived high morbidity, mortality, and resource utilization of these procedures. Second, presenting the evidence using standardized oncologic terminology applied to primary spine tumors was done with the goal of increasing awareness of the nuances associated with the surgical management of these rare tumors and to encourage broader use of appropriate terminology so that future studies would be based on a common language.

Study Design   A systematic review of the literature was performed with independent reviewers and standardized study selection criteria.

---

* Yamazaki T, McLoughlin GS, Patel S, Rhines LD, Fourney DR. Feasibility and safety of en bloc resection for primary spine tumors: A systematic review by the Spine Oncology Study Group. *Spine (Phila Pa 1976)*. 2009; 34(22 Suppl): S31–S38.

Sample Size   From the 89 studies initially identified, the 8 studies selected for review presented results on a combined total of 311 patients with regard to the effect of biopsy method and 300 comparing en bloc versus intralesional resection.

Follow-Up   Length of follow-up varied by study.

Inclusion/Exclusion Criteria   Studies were identified on the criteria that each reported more than 10 low-grade malignant tumors of the mobile spine and described oncologic staging criteria, biopsy technique, tissue margins, complications, and disease-free survival.

Intervention or Treatment Received   Several interventions were analyzed. The primary focus was to compare en bloc versus intralesional resection; the second focus was to compare percutaneous CT-guided biopsy versus open biopsy. In addition, some patients in the reported studies received radiation therapy either alone or in combination with either intralesional or en bloc resection.

Results   Evidence from the reviewed studies demonstrates that en bloc resection is associated with significantly improved continuous disease-free survival in patients where adequate margins were achieved at surgery. Achievement of long term (>5 year) disease-free survival is best achieved with en bloc resection. Both open biopsy and previously attempted intralesional resection are associated with decreased likelihood of achieving acceptable margins and decreased disease-free survival, and are therefore strongly discouraged. Use of en bloc resection techniques to achieve oncologically appropriate margins is possible when determined to be feasible based on Enneking and Weinstein, Boriani, Biagini (WBB) staging systems.[1,2] The safety of these aggressive operations was scrutinized and, not surprisingly, demonstrated a high rate of morbidity both from planned causes such as the sacrifice of nerve roots required to effect an en bloc removal of tumor, and from unplanned complications such as intraoperative hemorrhage, infection, wound breakdown, implant failure/spinal instability, and/or local recurrence. The risk of these complications was seen to be significantly higher in revision surgeries (i.e., after previous intralesional resection) and could be minimized when multidisciplinary surgical teams and specialized techniques (i.e., complex flap closure) were employed.

Study Limitations   While randomized, controlled trials comparing intralesional to en bloc resection would better answer these questions, they are not feasible given the rarity of these diseases, the variety of surgeon preferences and techniques, and challenges with patients accepting randomization between such radically different approaches. With randomized control trials (RCTs) and therefore meta-analyses precluded, this systematic review was utilized to maximize the grade of recommendation that could be derived from all the available evidence. The conditions studied are rare diseases, so even in combining these studies, low numbers of patients are reported. While the principles guiding these surgical techniques are standardized, the exact procedures performed are highly individualized and could make these data difficult to extrapolate. Additionally, postoperative treatments including radiation and/or chemotherapy are only marginally considered in this article, and their contribution to disease-free survival cannot be evaluated. Last, quality of life is not considered, so while this article can help answer whether it is feasible and safe to perform en bloc resection, the decision of whether or not it is worth pursuing this aggressive strategy, which requires weighing upfront morbidity against increased progression-free survival, must still be discussed with patients on an individual basis.

Relevant Studies   Advances in surgical approaches, anesthesia, and reconstructive techniques have made en bloc resection of spine tumors possible. Compared to intralesional resection, these techniques have improved disease-free survival and offer patients their best chance for cure. This article helps to establish the strategy of CT-guided, as opposed to open, biopsy followed by en bloc resection for primary spine tumors such as chordoma and chondrosarcoma. Performing these complex procedures results in improved oncologic outcome at the cost of increased but acceptable morbidity, especially when done in specialized centers. Using the Enneking and WBB classifications to stage tumors and guide treatment is shown to have moderate interobserver and near perfect intraobserver reliability but awaits prospective validation.[3] Since the publication of this article, several case series reporting an increasingly larger worldwide experience with en bloc resection have been reported. Several collaborative case series reporting large numbers of chordomas and chondrosarcomas of the sacrum and mobile spine treated at major international centers support the conclusions of this study: that these techniques, when feasible, provide the best oncologic outcome in terms of freedom from local progression. Interestingly, not all such[4–10] series report improvements in overall survival, which is somewhat paradoxical given that local recurrence typically affects survival. What is the explanation for this finding? Last, the optimal integration of focused radiation techniques with surgical resection of these lesions remains to be elucidated. A small case series with limited follow-up indicating that significant rates of disease-free survival can be achieved by combining less invasive surgery with focused radiation was recently reported.[11] How does this compare with radiation using heavy particles? Prospective evaluation with long-term follow-up will be necessary to answer these questions.

REFERENCES

1. Enneking WF, Spanier SS, Goodman MA. A system for the surgical staging of musculo-skeletal sarcoma. *Clinical Orthopaedics and Relat Res.* 1980; 153: 106–120.
2. Hart RA, Boriani S, Biagini R, Currier B, Weinstein JN. A system for surgical staging and management of spine tumors. A clinical outcome study of giant cell tumors of the spine. *Spine.* 1997; 22(15): 1773–1783.
3. Chan P, Boriani S, Fourney DR, et al. An assessment of the reliability of the Enneking and Weinstein-Boriani-Biagini classifications for staging of primary spinal tumors by the Spine Oncology Study Group. *Spine.* 2009; 34(4): 384–391.
4. Boriani S, Gasbarrini A, Bandiera S, Ghermandi R, Lador R. Predictors for surgical complications of en bloc resections in the spine: Review of 220 cases treated by the same team. *European Spine J.* 2016; 25(12): 3932–3941.
5. Boriani S, Gasbarrini A, Bandiera S, Ghermandi R, Lador R. En bloc resections in the spine—The experience of 220 cases over 25 years. *World Neurosurgery.* 2016.
6. Fisher CG, Versteeg AL, Dea N, et al. Surgical management of spinal chondrosarcomas. *Spine.* 2016; 41(8): 678–685.
7. Gokaslan ZL, Zadnik PL, Sciubba DM, et al. Mobile spine chordoma: Results of 166 patients from the AOSpine Knowledge Forum Tumor database. *J Neurosurg Spine.* 2016; 24(4): 644–651.
8. Hsieh PC, Gallia GL, Sciubba DM, et al. En bloc excisions of chordomas in the cervical spine: Review of five consecutive cases with more than 4-year follow-up. *Spine.* 2011; 36(24): E1581–1587.
9. Li D, Guo W, Tang X, Ji T, Zhang Y. Surgical classification of different types of en bloc resection for primary malignant sacral tumors. *European Spine J.* 2011; 20(12): 2275–2281.
10. Varga PP, Szoverfi Z, Fisher CG, et al. Surgical treatment of sacral chordoma: Prognostic variables for local recurrence and overall survival. *European Spine J.* 2015; 24(5): 1092–1101.
11. Lockney DT, Shub T, Hopkins B, et al. Spinal stereotactic body radiotherapy following intralesional curettage with separation surgery for initial or salvage chordoma treatment. *Neurosurgical Focus.* 2017; 42(1): E4.

CHAPTER 9

The Three-Column Spine and Its Significance in the Classification of Acute Thoracolumbar Spine Injuries*

Denis F. Spine 8(8):817–831, 1983

Reviewed by Daniel Mendelsohn and Marcel F. Dvorak

Research Question/Objective   Injuries of the thoracic and lumbar spine occur frequently. The purpose of this study was to build on the existing two-column model of the spine by proposing the existence of a third middle column. The contribution of the middle column to spinal stability in trauma was evaluated for different fracture types and injury mechanisms, and the association with neurological injury is described.

Study Design   A retrospective review of thoracic and lumbar spine injuries treated at the Ramsey Medical Center in St. Paul, Minnesota, and the Ottawa Civical Hospital in Ottawa, Canada, was conducted. Charts, operative notes, radiographs, myelograms, and CT scans were reviewed when available.

Sample Size   Four hundred and twelve thoracic and lumbar spine injuries were reviewed, of which 120 had operative notes and 53 had CT scans available.

Follow-Up   Average follow-up was 30.1 months.

Inclusion/Exclusion Criteria   Patients with metastatic fractures, severe osteoporosis, ankylosing spondylitis, bone tumors, and metabolic bone disease were excluded.

Intervention   One-third of patients were managed operatively; however, the purpose of the study was not to analyze different methods of treatment.

---

* Denis F. The three-column spine and its significance in the classification of acute thoracolumbar spinal injuries. *Spine.* 1983; 8(8): 817–831.

Results A new biomechanical model of the spine was proposed involving a middle column formed by the posterior longitudinal ligament, the posterior annulus fibrosus, and the posterior wall of the vertebral body. The contribution of the three columns to spinal stability was evaluated for four fracture types: compression, burst, seat-belt type, and fracture dislocation. Review of 197 compression fractures in 136 patients led to the conclusion that the middle column is intact in this type of injury. These patients were all neurologically intact, and the spinal canal was not narrowed in 10 patients who had CT scans. Burst fractures occurred in 59 cases and were attributed to failure of the anterior and middle columns by axial loading. Thirty CT scans in this subgroup demonstrated fracture of the posterior vertebral body wall leading to retropulsion and varying degrees of canal stenosis. The relationship between degree of narrowing and neurological injury depended on the location of the injury (spinal cord, conus medullaris, or cauda equina) and the corresponding space available for the neural elements. Burst fractures were subdivided into 5 types based on the fracture pattern, although their clinical importance was not defined. Seat-belt injuries, which occurred in 19 cases, were characterized by failure of the middle and posterior column with varying degrees on anterior column collapse; classic bony chance fractures are included in this category. Seat-belt injuries were subdivided into one- and two-level lesions. Fracture dislocation involved failure of all three spinal columns under compression. Tension, rotational and shearing forces was observed in 67 cases. These fractures were subdivided into flexion rotation, shear, and flexion-distraction subtypes.

The association between the four thoracic and lumbar fracture types and neurologic injury were analyzed. All compression and seat-belt type injuries were either neurologically intact or had concomitant unrelated peripheral nerve-type injuries. Approximately half of patients with burst fractures and three-quarters with flexion distraction type injuries had neurological deficits.

Denis defined three degrees of instability, based on the presence of mechanical only (first degree), neurological only (second degree) or both mechanical and neurological instability (third degree).

Study Limitations The major limitations of this study are its retrospective design and primitive radiographic evaluation. This retrospective study is limited by selection bias and information bias affecting the generalizability of results to other populations. Only 53 patients had cross-sectional imaging with CT scans, and the study was conducted in the pre-magnetic resonance imaging (MRI) era, limiting the radiographic evaluation to bony fracture pattern analysis, with less information about the disco-ligamentous structures and neurological elements. The study did not investigate the reproducibility and reliability of the classification scheme; however, subsequent investigations found interobserver reliability to be modest (kappa = 0.6) for major fracture type classification.[1]

The study describes subtypes for compression, burst, seat-belt type, and fracture-dislocations, but these subgroupings are of unclear clinical significance (i.e., no explicit description of which fractures are unstable). The simplification of the fracture types is valuable; however, some fracture patterns are not included, and the contribution of the ligamentous structures to spinal stability is not addressed comprehensively. The degree of kyphosis, which was subsequently demonstrated to have importance in the operative management of the thoracolumbar injuries, is also not incorporated in the classification.[2] Similarly, the role of the sternal-rib complex in spinal stability is not addressed; the sternal-rib complex is labeled by other authors as the *fourth column* of the spine.[3] Although the relationship of the fracture types and neurological deficits is explored, the presence of neurological injury is not incorporated in the classification system. The role of the middle column to spinal stability in the different fracture types is well described, although no specific management recommendations are made. Which fractures require surgical stabilization and the optimal methods for stabilizing these fracture types are not specified. Combined anterior and middle column injuries such as in burst fractures are suggested to be unstable; however, many burst fractures are successfully managed conservatively with or without bracing.[4]

Relevant Studies A decade later, Magerl and colleagues developed the AO Spine Classification System[5] based on analysis 1445 thoracic and lumbar injuries. The classification provides a more detailed description of fracture patterns and encompasses a larger variety of thoracolumbar injuries. The CT findings for the fracture types are described in more detail compared to the Denis three-column model. However, the classification is cumbersome and has poor interobserver reliability (kappa = 0.34), and the neurological status of the patient is not considered. In 2005, Vaccaro and colleagues developed the Thoracolumbar Injury Classification and Severity Score (TLICS), which included integrity of the posterior ligamentous complex and neurological status in addition to fracture morphology in the classification.[1] The TLICS system also provides recommendations on whether the fractures should be managed operatively or nonoperatively but does not specify the optimal surgical approach. The shortcomings of the TLICS system were later addressed with a new AOSpine Thoracolumbar Spine Injury Classification System in 2013.[6]

REFERENCES

1. Vaccaro AR, Lehman RA Jr., Hurlbert RJ, et al. A new classification of thoracolumbar injuries: The importance of injury morphology, the integrity of the posterior ligamentous complex, and neurologic status. *Spine.* 2005; 30: 2325–2333.
2. Farcy JP, Weidenbaum M, Glassman SD. Sagittal index in management of thoracolumbar burst fractures. *Spine.* 1990; 15: 958–965.

3. Berg EE. The sternal-rib complex: A possible fourth column in thoracic spine fractures. *Spine*. 1993; 18: 1916–1919.
4. Bailey CS, Urquhart JC, Dvorak MF, et al. Orthosis versus no orthosis for the treatment of thoracolumbar burst fractures without neurologic injury: A multicenter prospective randomized equivalence trial. *Spine J*. 2014; 14: 2557–2564.
5. Magerl F, Aebi M, Gertzbein SD, Harms J, Nazarian S. A comprehensive classification of thoracic and lumbar injuries. *Eur Spine J*. 1994; 3: 184–201.
6. Vaccaro AR, Oner C, Kepler CK, et al. AOSpine thoracolumbar spine injury classification system: Fracture description, neurological status, and key modifiers. *Spine*. 2013; 38: 2028–2037.

A Randomized, Controlled Trial of Methylprednisolone or Naloxone in the Treatment of Acute Spinal-Cord Injury*

Bracken MB, et al. N Engl J Med 322(20):1405–1411, 1990

Reviewed by Christopher S. Ahuja and Michael G. Fehlings

Research Question/Objective The National Acute Spinal Cord Injury Study[1] (NASCIS I) found no difference in motor or sensory outcomes between IV methylprednisolone (MPSS) at 100 mg × 10 days and 1000 mg × 10 days; however, animal data emerging in parallel with the study suggested that both doses were below the theoretical therapeutic threshold (30 mg/kg bolus).[2,3] This study (NASCIS II) was undertaken to assess the efficacy of a higher-dose MPSS protocol versus placebo. A third group receiving naloxone hydrochloride, an opiate-receptor antagonist, was also added after strong preclinical data found improved neurological recovery with early treatment.[4–6] The primary goal of this study was to establish the clinical efficacy and safety of IV MPSS and IV naloxone in acute spinal cord injury (SCI).

Study Design A prospective, multicenter, placebo-controlled clinical trial of patients with acute SCI randomized within 12 hours of their injury. All treatments and assessments were performed in a blinded fashion. Neurological outcome scores were standardized across sites and calculated as sums of the motor grade across myotomes and sensory function across dermatomes bilaterally.

Sample Size A total of 487 patients were randomized to methylprednisolone ($n = 162$), naloxone ($n = 154$), or placebo ($n = 171$).

Follow-Up Of surviving patients, neurological examinations were completed in 97.9% at 6 weeks and 96.5% at 6 months. Mortality data was obtained on all patients.

---
* Bracken MB, et al. A randomized, controlled trial of methylprednisolone or naloxone in the treatment of acute spinal-cord injury. Results of the Second National Acute Spinal Cord Injury Study. *N Engl J Med.* 1990; 322(20): 1405–1411. doi:10.1056/NEJM199005173222001.

Inclusion/Exclusion Criteria   Consenting patients aged 13 or older who were randomized within 12 hours of their injury were included in this study. Patients were excluded if they had (1) nerve root or cauda equina injuries only, (2) gunshot wounds, or (3) life-threatening morbidity; or they were (4) pregnant, (5) addicted to narcotics, (6) receiving maintenance steroids prior to presentation, (7) deemed difficult to follow up; or they had received prior to admission more than (8) 100 mg of MPSS or its equivalent, or (9) 1 mg of naloxone.

Intervention or Treatment Received   Due to differences in the appearance and solubility of naloxone and MPSS, each drug required its own placebo. Patients received either (1) naloxone placebo and MPSS, (2) naloxone and MPSS placebo, or (3) naloxone placebo and MPSS placebo. No patient received both naloxone and MPSS. Drugs were administered according to one of three possible schedules based on the patients' calculated body surface area to approximate an IV MPSS dose of 30 mg/kg bolus + 5.4 mg/kg/hr × 23 hours maintenance or an IV naloxone dose of 5.4 mg/kg bolus + 4.0 mg/kg/hr × 23 hours maintenance.

Results   The majority of patients were male (84.0%), aged 13–34 (69.3%), and presented with complete injuries (59.2%); 47.1% were quadriplegic and 32.9% were paraplegic at admission. The most common causes of injury were motor vehicle accidents (42.3%) and falls (19.5%). The mean time from injury to admission was 3.1 ± 2.6 hours and from injury to bolus dose was 8.7 ± 3.0 hours. There were no meaningful differences in admission characteristics between the three treatment groups.

The authors hypothesized a priori that time to drug administration was critically important. As a result, the analysis of neurological outcomes was stratified according to the injury to treatment time (≤ 8 hours versus >8 hours) and adjusted for injury severity (complete versus incomplete). All data reported was from the right side of the body. At 6 weeks postinjury, patients treated with MPSS had greater improvements in their motor score (10.6 versus 7.2; $p = 0.048$), light touch sensation (6.3 versus 2.5; $p = 0.034$), and pinprick sensation (7.8 versus 4.8; $p = 0.061$) compared with the placebo group. Patients treated with naloxone at any time or MPSS after 8 hours did not show a significant change. At 6 months postinjury, the group receiving MPSS within 8 hours demonstrated further recovery of motor (16.0 versus 11.2; $p = 0.033$), light touch (8.9 versus 4.3; $p = 0.030$), and pinprick (16.0 versus 11.2; $p = 0.016$) compared to placebo (Table 10.1). It is important to note that these effects were found in patients with both complete and incomplete injuries. Naloxone and MPSS after 8 hours had no significant effect. When the analysis was repeated including only patients receiving treatments in accordance with the study protocol, the effects of early MPSS were even more substantial across motor (17.2 versus 10.7; $p = 0.011$), light touch (9.8 versus 4.6; $p = 0.020$), and pinprick (12.9 versus 5.9; $p = 0.001$) function.

Table 10.1 Change in Neurologic Measures 6 Weeks and 6 Months after Injury in Patients Who Received the Study Drug within 8 Hours of Injury[a]

Category of Injury and Measure[b]	6 Weeks			6 Months		
	Methylprednisolone	Naloxone	Placebo	Methylprednisolone	Naloxone	Placebo
Change in Score (p Value)						
Plegic with total sensory loss						
No. of patients	47	37	46	45	34	44
Motor	6.2 (0.021)	3.2 (0.394)	1.3 (R)	10.5 (0.019)	7.5 (0.254)	4.2 (R)
Pinprick	5.9 (0.062)	3.0 (0.690)	2.2 (R)	9.4 (0.028)	4.2 (0.947)	4.0 (R)
Touch	6.8 (0.051)	3.7 (0.622)	2.6 (R)	9.7 (0.050)	7.1 (0.374)	4.7 (R)
Plegic with partial sensory loss						
No. of patients	5	12	6	5	11	6
Motor	14.4 (0.564)	14.1 (0.447)	18.0 (R)	23.0 (0.652)	28.9 (0.711)	26.5 (R)
Pinprick	11.8 (0.168)	13.9 (0.037)	4.0 (R)	11.6 (0.803)	18.4 (0.152)	9.8 (R)
Touch	4.4 (0.515)	7.1 (0.204)	0.3 (R)	0.0 (0.479)	13.5 (0.181)	5.2 (R)
Plegic with variable sensory loss						
No. of patients	14	12	17	12	11	17
Motor	18.3 (0.054)	12.7 (0.635)	10.8 (R)	24.3 (0.018)	14.5 (0.738)	12.9 (R)
Pinprick	10.7 (0.368)	8.2 (0.844)	7.5 (R)	14.3 (0.133)	9.6 (0.633)	7.5 (R)
Touch	3.8 (0.518)	6.1 (0.237)	1.2 (R)	7.6 (0.174)	6.2 (0.285)	1.0 (R)

Reproduced from Bracken MB et al, *N Engl J Med*. 1990; 322, 1405–1411. With permission.
[a] R denotes reference value. The *p* values were determined from analysis of variance.
[b] Scores for motor function range from 0 to 70. Scores for sensations of pinprick and touch each range from 29 to 87.

Complication rates were similar between the three groups; however, a nonsignificant trend toward increased wound infection (7.1% versus 3.6%) and gastrointestinal bleeding (4.5% versus 3.0%) was seen with MPSS versus placebo. Morality rates were similar among all treatment groups (~6%).

Study Limitations   The key results of this study were demonstrated in the subgroup analysis instead of the primary analysis, making the findings more controversial. In particular, whether the 8-hour stratification time point was in fact a priori has been a source of significant controversy. As well, the statistical analysis applies over 50 individual t-tests and omnibus tests to compare treatment groups without correcting for multiple comparisons. This introduces a significant risk of Type I error. Furthermore, several study parameters, including neurological outcome, are likely nonparametric, making ANOVA and t-tests less appropriate. Another common criticism of NASCIS II is the clinical significance of a 5-point motor score improvement; however, patients do consistently report that even small improvements in critical myotomes (e.g., grip, wrist extension, deltoid function) can have a profound effect on their quality of life and independence (e.g., feeding, grooming).

Relevant Studies   NASCIS I ($n = 330$) found no difference in sensory or motor scores with 10 days of MPSS but did find an increase in wound infection rates ($p = 0.01$).[1] Concurrent animal studies suggested, however, that even the 1000 mg dose failed to reach the therapeutic threshold, and thus the short, high-dose NASCIS II protocol was developed.[2,3]

After NASCIS II, Otani and colleagues published a 1996 report of the only trial to directly study high-dose MPSS administered within 8 hours of injury. While they did report improved neurological outcomes with treatment, the study was not blinded and participants were pseudo-randomized to experimental groups, thereby limiting strong conclusions.[7] In 1997, the multicenter, prospective, double-blind NASCIS III ($n = 499$) trial was published comparing 24 versus 48 hours of MPSS without a placebo group. Patients receiving the 48-hour protocol had greater motor recovery than the 24-hour group at 6 weeks (12.5 versus 7.6; $p = 0.04$) and 6 months (17.6 versus 11.2; $p = 0.01$) but only in the subgroup receiving the drug from 3 to 8 hours postinjury. The longer protocol, however, also showed a trend toward increased severe pneumonia (5.8% versus 2.6%) and sepsis (2.6% versus 0.6%).[8,9] These results led to a joint 2002 American Association of Neurological Surgeons (AANS)/Congress of Neurological Surgeons (CNS) guideline suggesting 24 to 48 hours of IV MPSS be considered as an option for acute SCI.[10] Despite no new prospective randomized data and a Cochrane systematic review in favor of early MPSS (mean weighted difference = 4.06 [0.58–7.55]),[11] a 2013 AANS/CNS guideline recommended against using MPSS for SCI, sparking significant debate.[12] The 2017 AOSpine guideline developed by an international, interdisciplinary expert committee suggested that

24 hours of IV MPSS be considered as an option for patients with acute, non-penetrating SCI within 8 hours of injury and no significant medical comorbidities.[13] The guideline will also recommend against the 48-hour infusion due to increased complications. This differentiation between 24 and 48 hours of MPSS will help to clarify the discrepancy between the 2002 and 2013 AANS/CNS guidelines.

ACKNOWLEDGMENTS

Thank you to Madeleine O'Higgins for copyediting this work.

REFERENCES

1. Bracken MB, et al. Efficacy of methylprednisolone in acute spinal cord injury. *JAMA.* 1984; 251: 45–52.
2. Hall ED, Braughler, JM. Glucocorticoid mechanisms in acute spinal cord injury: A review and therapeutic rationale. *Surg Neurol.* 1982; 18: 320–327.
3. Braughler JM, Hall ED. Lactate and pyruvate metabolism in injured cat spinal cord before and after a single large intravenous dose of methylprednisolone. *J Neurosurg.* 1983; 59, 256–261, doi:10.3171/jns.1983.59.2.0256.
4. Faden AI, Jacobs TP, Holaday JW. Opiate antagonist improves neurologic recovery after spinal injury. *Science.* 1981; 211: 493–494.
5. Faden AI, Jacobs TP, Mougey E, Holaday JW. Endorphins in experimental spinal injury: Therapeutic effect of naloxone. *Ann Neurol.* 1981; 10: 326–332, doi:10.1002/ana.410100403.
6. Young W, Flamm ES, Demopoulos HB, Tomasula JJ, DeCrescito V. Effect of naloxone on posttraumatic ischemia in experimental spinal contusion. *J Neurosurg.* 1981; 55: 209–219, doi:10.3171/jns.1981.55.2.0209.
7. Otani KAH, Kadoya S, Nakagawa H, Ikata T, Tominaga S. Beneficial effect of methylprednisolone sodium succinate in the treatment of acute spinal cord injury. *Sekitsui Sekizui J.* 1996; 7: 633.
8. Bracken MB, et al. Administration of methylprednisolone for 24 or 48 hours or tirilazad mesylate for 48 hours in the treatment of acute spinal cord injury: Results of the Third National Acute Spinal Cord Injury Randomized Controlled Trial. National Acute Spinal Cord Injury Study. *JAMA.* 1997; 277: 1597–1604.
9. Bracken MB, et al. Methylprednisolone or tirilazad mesylate administration after acute spinal cord injury: 1-year follow up. Results of the third National Acute Spinal Cord Injury randomized controlled trial. *J Neurosurg.* 1998; 89: 699–706, doi:10.3171/jns.1998.89.5.0699.
10. Hadley MN, et al. Guidelines for the management of acute cervical spine and spinal cord injuries. *Clin Neurosurg.* 2002; 49: 407–498.
11. Bracken, MB. Steroids for acute spinal cord injury. *Cochrane Database Syst Rev.* 2012; 1: CD001046, doi:10.1002/14651858.CD001046.pub2.
12. Resnick DK. Updated guidelines for the management of acute cervical spine and spinal cord injury. *Neurosurgery.* 2013; 72(Suppl 2): 1, doi:10.1227/NEU.0b013e318276ee7e.
13. Fehlings MG, et al. A clinical practice guideline for the management of patients with acute spinal cord injury: recommendations on the use of methylprednisolone sodium succinate. *Global Spine J.* 2017; 7(3_suppl): 203S–211S, doi:10.1177/2195568217703085.

Methylprednisolone for Acute Spinal Cord Injury: An Inappropriate Standard of Care*

Hurlbert R. John. J Neurosurg 93:1–7, 2000

Reviewed by Bornali Kundu and Gregory W. J. Hawryluk

Research Question/Objective   Acute spinal cord injury (SCI) is a devastating condition that has limited treatment options. Intravenous methylprednisolone sodium succinate (MPSS) may be a potential treatment based on its anti-inflammatory mechanisms of action. Several randomized controlled trials have studied the effects of MPSS administration in SCI patients. The National Acute Spinal Cord Injury Studies (NASCIS)[1–3] were the highest quality studies that assessed whether MPSS administration was associated with improved outcomes in SCI patients. Following the publication of NASCIS 2, MPSS administration within 8 hours of acute SCI became a standard of care and was widely adopted around the world.

This landmark paper published by Hurlbert in 2000 critically examined the literature supporting MPSS use for acute SCI and raised important questions about whether MPSS administration truly should be a standard of care. The author asserts that such standards should be supported by data derived from well-designed, randomized, controlled trials. Results must show internal consistency and be produced by appropriate statistical methods. Finally, the results should be meaningful to the patient and be reproducible. Hurlbert asserts that the NASCIS studies did not meet these criteria. The legacy of his influential paper has been a gradual decline in the use of MPSS for acute SCI and loss of its *standard of care* status.

Study Design   Note that this article is not a trial itself but is a critical reanalysis and independent interpretation of the published data for NASCIS 2 and 3 and their respective 1-year follow-up studies. Relevant data from these trials were converted from tabular form and plotted on a single time line. Data related to the other drugs examined in the NASCIS studies were not considered in the author's reinterpretation.

---

* Hurlbert RJ. Methylprednisolone for acute spinal cord injury: An inappropriate standard of care. *J Neurosurg.* 2000; 93: 1–7.

Sample Size The sample size of NASCIS 2 was 487 patients and of NASCIS 3 was 499 patients.

Follow-Up Both NASCIS 2 and 3 studies reported 6-month follow-up in the initial publications; 1-year follow-up data was subsequently published.[4,5]

Inclusion/Exclusion Criteria Patients with acute SCI were included in the analyses. Exclusion criteria for NASCIS 2 and 3 varied.

Intervention or Treatment Received MPSS for the treatment of acute SCI.

Results The criticism presented by Hurlbert (2000) is broken down by the above-mentioned criteria delineating a standard of care. He finds both NASCIS 2 and 3 trials to be well-designed and well-executed randomized controlled trials with good follow-up rates. NASCIS 2 tested whether the effects of MPSS vary with time of administration and severity of injury. One of the author's major points of contention is that the time point chosen for early administration was, in his opinion, not clearly defined a priori. The analyses divided patients into two categories, drug administration within 8 hours of injury and after that time. The author points out that there is no cited literature to support this time-point cutoff, and suggests that the investigators most likely chose the time point that showed favorable results after testing all possible time points. Similarly, in NASCIS 3, the patients were grouped into those who received MPSS before or after 3 hours. Again, Hurlbert points out this time point may have been arbitrarily chosen post hoc. See the counterargument posed by Bracken (2000).[6]

Motor function was measured in terms of a numerical motor score based on strength in predefined muscle groups of the arm or leg for right and left sides. However, the reported results included only data from the right-sided motor function, while bilateral sensory function is reported. There is a summary statement in the methods of NASCIS 2 indicating the investigators repeated the entire study's analyses using left-sided motor scores and produced the same results, but Hurlbert points out that there was no need to omit left-sided motor data, since bilateral sensory data were included. In the original trial, the results were grouped by functional status of the patient including having complete motor and sensory deficits, complete motor and partial sensory deficits, and finally partial motor and sensory loss. Hurlbert reports such comparisons are invalid due to low numbers within groups (e.g., $n = 12$) that do not provide meaningful statistical comparisons.

The author argues that the results for both NASCIS 2 and 3 studies fail to be compelling or to justify MPSS use as a standard of care. He states that the primary outcome of NASCIS 2 did not show a difference in motor or sensory outcomes between MPSS (drug given at any time point) and placebo groups at the 1-year mark. He then reports that, while patients who received MPSS within 8 hours of injury did have statistically significant improvements in motor and sensory function, the small difference in improvement between groups in NASCIS 2 may not be meaningful to a patient. For NASCIS 3, he produces motor or sensory score versus time plots for the 24 hours versus 48 hours MPSS administration groups. He reports there are no significant differences between groups at 1 year. He also points out that the Functional Independence Measure (FIM score; a proxy for clinically meaningful recovery) used in NASCIS 3 does not show significant differences between MPSS administration groups 1 year out.

Last, the authors of NASCIS 3 report results with and without intention to treat. Hurlbert points out that clinical trials should always be reported with intention to treat; not doing so otherwise inflates the effects of any one group. Furthermore, the difference in *p*-values between these two analyses in NASCIS 3 is nearly an order of magnitude different for a difference carried by 8 patients, suggesting that the data are statistically *unstable* and thus lacking internal reliability. He points out that, when one drops the *non-compliers* in the 24-hour MPSS administration group, the group fares worse than when one includes the *non-compliers*, implying that not taking the medication helps motor function, which does not make sense. Additionally, NASCIS 3 was not designed to interrogate whether MPSS is more effective at treating SCI compared to placebo, which is an inherent weakness of the trial. Finally, he points out that both studies did not control for multiple comparisons and that, while not significant, MPSS administration is associated with higher rates of complications.

Thus, despite having Class I evidence, the data are not compelling enough to support MPSS administration as a standard of care for SCI patients.

Study Limitations   Hurlbert did not have access to the NASCIS datasets, making many of his arguments speculative. Accordingly, Hurlbert's review has been criticized for reproducing a statistically *summarized version* of the trial data that is lacking information with regard to patient baseline function and other sources of variance.[6] His critical analysis and opinions have been viewed as hypercritical by many. Indeed, he holds the NASCIS studies to a higher standard than what existed at the time the studies were conceived and published—NASCIS 2 was published 10 years prior to his critique. Nonetheless the critiques offered by Hurlbert have been extremely influential and have helped to improve the design and interpretation of subsequent studies.

Relevant Studies   Several additional studies are important to consider in the MPSS debate, although these studies provide lower-quality evidence than the NASCIS studies. Otani et al. (1994), a multicenter study in Japan, used the NASICS 2 MPSS protocol compared to placebo and found improved motor scores at 6-month follow-up.[7] Petitjean et al. (1998), a single center trial from France, also used the NASCIS 2 trial MPSS regimen and found no difference between placebo and MPSS.[8] A recent study from a Canadian database found baseline level of injury and cervical injury to be significant predictors of functional recovery. MPSS administration did not improve functional recovery when those two measures were used as covariates.[9] Notably, the timing of the neurological exam was not standardized and could bias the results.

A Cochrane analysis published in 2002 and revised in 2012 is supportive of MPSS administration in SCI, demonstrating significant motor improvement and a reduction in mortality with MPSS administration.[10] Notably, these meta-analyses were authored by the lead author of the NASCIS studies. Another recent meta-analysis addresses this question and includes all relevant randomized controlled trials and pooled results from a number of observational studies. This review concluded that available evidence does not support routine administration of MPSS.[11]

On the heels of Hurlbert's landmark paper, the 2002 acute SCI guidelines effectively removed MPSS as a standard of care, recommending MPSS as only a treatment option. The controversial 2013 acute SCI guidelines[12] generated a Level 1 recommendation against the use of MPSS despite little change in the available literature. Our recent survey finds that SCI patients thought the small benefits inherent to MPSS were very important to them and they expressed little concern with the side effects inherent to MPSS.[13] We believe that, when possible, patients should be given greater autonomy in deciding whether or not MPSS is administered, although this is not possible for many acutely injured patients.

REFERENCES

1. Bracken MB, Collins WF, Freeman DF, et al. Efficacy of methylprednisolone in acute spinal cord injury. *JAMA*. 1984; 251(1): 45–52. doi:10.1001/jama.1984.03340250025015.
2. Bracken M, Shepard M, Collins W, et al. A randomized, controlled trial of methylprednisolone or naloxone in the treatment of acute spinal cord injury. *N Engl J Med*. 1990; 322(20): 1405–1411.
3. Bracken MB, Shepard MJ, Holford TR, et al. Administration of methylprednisolone for 24 or 48 hours or tirilazad mesylate for 48 hours in the treatment of acute spinal cord injury. Results of the Third National Acute Spinal Cord Injury Randomized Controlled Trial. National Acute Spinal Cord Injury. *JAMA*. 1997; 277(20): 1597–1604.
4. Bracken MB, Shepard MJ, Hellenbrand KG, et al. Methylprednisolone and neurological function 1 year after spinal cord injury. Results of the National Acute Spinal Cord Injury Study. *J Neurosurg*. 1985; 63(5): 704–713.
5. Bracken MB, Shepard MJ, Collins WF, et al. Methylprednisolone or naloxone treatment after acute spinal cord injury: 1-year follow-up data. *J Neurosurg*. 1992; 76(1): 23–31.
6. Bracken M. Letters: Methylprednisolone and spinal cord injury. *J Neurosurg*. 2000; 93: 175–179.
7. Otani K, Abe H, Kadoya S. Beneficial effect of methylprednisolone sodium succinate in the treatment of acute spinal cord injury (translation of Japanese). *Sekitsui Sekizui*. 1994; 7: 633–647.

8. Petitjean M, Pointillart V, Dixmerias F, et al. Traitement medicamenteux de la lesion medullaire traumatique au stade aigu. *Ann Fr d-anesthesie Reanim.* 1998; 17: 115–122.
9. Evaniew N, Noonan VK, Fallah N, et al. Methylprednisolone for the treatment of patients with acute spinal cord injuries: A propensity score-matched cohort Study from a Canadian multi-center spinal cord injury registry. *J Neurotrauma.* 2015; 1683: 1674–1683.
10. Bracken M. Steroids for acute spinal cord injury. *Cochrane Database Syst Rev.* 2012; (1): 1–15.
11. Evaniew N, Belley-Cote EP, Fallah N, Noonan V, Rivers CS, Dvorak MF. Methylprednisolone for the treatment of patients with acute spinal cord injuries: A systematic review and meta-analysis 1. *J Neurotrauma.* 2015; 481(1557-9042): 468–481.
12. Hurlbert RJ, Hadley MN, Walters BC, et al. Pharmacological therapy for acute spinal cord injury. *Neurosurgery.* 2013; 72(Suppl.2): 93–105.
13. Bowers CA, Kundu B, Rosenbluth J, Hawryluk GWJ. Patients with Spinal Cord Injuries Favor Administration of Methylprednisolone. *PLoS One.* (2016); 11(1): e0145991.

CHAPTER 12

Fractures of the Odontoid Process of the Axis*

Anderson LD, D'Alonzo RT. J Bone Joint Surg Am 56(8):1663–1674, 1974

Reviewed by Joseph S. Butler and Andrew P. White

Research Question/Objective Odontoid fractures account for 9%–15% of cervical spine fractures in the adult population.[1] These injuries can be associated with a high rate of morbidity and mortality, regardless of treatment method. Several factors account for this, including nonunion comorbidities in elderly patients, and complications from the use of restrictive bracing and/or surgery. The purpose of this study was to report the results of a large series of fractures of the odontoid process, examine the effects of different treatment strategies on outcome, and develop a classification system to characterize common fracture patterns and guide future treatment strategies.

Study Design A retrospective review of the management and outcome of a large series of fractures of the odontoid process of the axis treated at the Campbell Clinic and City of Memphis Hospital over an 18-year period.

Sample Size Sixty patients were treated at the Campbell Clinic and City of Memphis Hospital between January 1954 and June 1972. Nine patients had inadequate follow-up (<6 months), 2 patients died within 1 week of injury, leaving 49 patients with a follow-up of a minimum 6 months.

Follow-Up Mean follow-up of 22 months (minimum 6 months).

Inclusion/Exclusion Criteria Eligibility criteria for the study included fractures of the odontoid process of the axis with a minimum follow-up of 6 months.

Intervention Surgical treatment and nonsurgical immobilization.

Results In this series (*n* = 49), the mean age was 40.7 years (range 3–76 years). The mechanisms of injury included motor vehicle accidents (35 out of 49),

* Anderson LD, D'Alonzo RT. Fractures of the odontoid process of the axis. *J Bone Joint Surg Am.* 1974; 56(8): 1663–1674.

falls (10 out of 49), and assault involving force applied to the back of head (4 out of 49). Associated injuries included cerebral contusions (12 out of 49), extremity fractures (10 out of 49), facial bone fractures (4 out of 49), and concurrent cervical spine fractures (4 out of 49).

Fractures were classified into three fracture patterns based on the anatomic location of the fracture line. Type I being an oblique avulsion-type fracture through the tip of the odontoid process, Type II being a fracture at the junction of the odontoid process and the body of the C2 vertebra, and Type III being a fracture extending into the cancellous portion of the body of the C2 vertebra. Fractures were further classified as nondisplaced or displaced.

There were two Type I fractures: Both were nondisplaced, were treated in collar or brace, and had no problems following treatment. The authors considered this to be a stable fracture pattern and advised treatment with immobilization alone.

There were 32 Type II fractures: 14 were nondisplaced and 18 were displaced (≥2 mm on lateral radiograph). All 14 nondisplaced fractures were treated by traction (head halter or tongs) for 6 weeks, followed by bracing, of which 9 united at a mean of 6.4 months and 5 developed nonunion. Of the 18 displaced fractures, 10 had primary C1-C2 posterior wiring and fusion, with 9 successfully uniting and 1 case on nonunion despite a solid posterior fusion; 8 were treated by traction (Crutchfield tongs) for 6 weeks followed by bracing, of which 5 united at a mean of 5.6 months and 3 developed nonunion. The authors considered this type of displaced fracture to be unstable, frequently becoming further displaced. With a 36% nonunion rate in those treated conservatively, primary fusion was recommended as the treatment of choice for this fracture pattern. It was proposed that conservatively treated patients progressing to nonunion should have surgical fusion performed to prevent late myelopathy.

There were 15 Type III fractures: 5 were nondisplaced and 10 were displaced. Of the 5 nondisplaced fractures, 4 were treated in traction followed by bracing and uniting at a mean of 5.5 months, 1 was treated with primary C1-C2 wiring and fusion and united by 12 weeks. Of the 10 displaced fractures, 9 were treated by traction followed by a brace or cast, of which 8 united in a satisfactory position at a mean of 4 months and 1 was a delayed presentation at 5 weeks after injury and treated in a collar or brace for 8 months; 1 patient had a primary fusion that united but was complicated by a postoperative infection that resolved by 6 months and required wire removal. The authors proposed that the large cancellous surface of the body of C2 contributes significantly to the greater than 90% union rate in this fracture pattern, with primary fusion being reserved only for cases of established nonunion.

Five children were treated during the study period. One was a 3-year-old who died in the first week after injury and was excluded from the study. The other four children who were followed up were aged between 3 and 6 years, none had any neurological findings, three were treated in traction for 6 weeks followed by Minerva cast (two Type II and one Type III fractures) and united at a mean of 4 months; 1 had a primary C1-C2 wiring and fusion (Type II fracture) that resulted in graft resorption and wire breakage but ultimately united in a satisfactory position. The authors felt that odontoid fractures in the pediatric population were physeal fractures and should be given the opportunity to unite with conservative treatment, with fusion reserved for cases of nonunion.

There was a low mortality rate in this series: two of the 60 patients originally identified died shortly after their injuries, with the odontoid fracture not considered to have contributed directly to their death. Early neurological deficits were present in 15 of the 60 initially treated patients (25%). These findings were minor in 10 patients, and only 5 patients had serious neurological involvement. Only two patients had disabling neurological problems after treatment.

There were 18 cervical fusions performed in this series, either as primary treatment or for established nonunion. Sixteen successful fusions were achieved after the first operation. Fusion of the first cervical vertebra to the second was considered adequate in the vast majority of patients, as primary treatment or to treat nonunion. The authors suggested that the occiput should be included only in the setting of a fracture or congenital deficiency in the ring of the first cervical vertebra. The third cervical vertebra should be included only if there is a fracture of the posterior elements of the second cervical vertebra.

Study Limitations   This early study examining the treatment and outcome of fractures of the odontoid process of the axis has a number of significant limitations that must be considered. The retrospective design likely has several inherent flaws, such as selection bias, misclassification and information bias, leading to inaccuracies in establishing the true incidence and mortality rates for this particular injury. The inclusion of patients 3–6 years of age with those greater than 65 years of age is inappropriate, due to differing physiology and coexisting morbidities affecting clinical decision making. The assessment of fracture union based solely on dynamic radiographic imaging, as opposed to the current *gold standard* of computed tomography (CT) scanning, is a significant weakness when drawing conclusions for current treatment strategies. The lack of standardization of the surgical and conservative management approaches makes it difficult to draw treatment-specific conclusions, and the lack of an agreed bracing protocol also raises concerns about treatment duration and compliance. The surgical decision making in this series appears to be based on individual surgeon preference as opposed to an agreed rationale. Furthermore, the neurological involvement is poorly delineated, with a lack of objective clinical and functional data or use of validated scoring systems. The lack of modern imaging modalities, such as magnetic resonance imaging (MRI), also weakens the relevance to modern practice, particularly since treatment decisions were made with the goal of preventing late myelopathy.

Relevant Studies   The classification system proposed in this study remains in widespread use, defining the natural history of odontoid fractures and facilitating improved treatment strategies. In particular, the distinction between Type II and Type III fractures has led to differing treatment strategies for each fracture. The natural history of Type II fracture has demonstrated a nonunion rate of 26%–85%,[2-4] due to considerably less trabecular bone at the base of the odontoid and the distractive forces from the apical ligament, contributing to an unfavorable healing potential.[5] The dens is surrounded by synovial cavities, resulting in diminished periosteal blood supply to Type II fractures. Consequently, it has been suggested that Type II injuries must be managed surgically to avoid late complications.[6] Conversely, nonsurgical bracing has remained the mainstay of management of stable Type III odontoid fractures, which have demonstrated high healing rates.[2]

The classification system presented has demonstrated limitations, with only fair interrater and intrarater reliability between spine surgeons and neuroradiologists.[7] Evaluation of plain radiographs resulted in kappa coefficients for interobserver and intraobserver agreement of 0.30 and 0.25, respectively, with significantly improved agreement achieved with the use of reformatted CT (interobserver, 0.46; intraobserver, 0.56). Therefore, it is agreed that substantial variability exists in the use of this classification system, even with the most experienced specialists.

A modification to the classification system was proposed to address some of these limitations.[8] This treatment-oriented classification system proposed three subtypes to stratify the Type II fracture pattern: Type IIA with a transverse fracture pattern and demonstrating <1 mm of displacement, Type IIB with an oblique fracture pattern extending from the anterosuperior to the posteroinferior portion of the dens, and Type IIIC beginning anteroinferiorly and extending posterosuperiorly and associated with significant anterior comminution. With the use of this Type II fracture subclassification, it was proposed to treat Type IIA fractures with external immobilization, Type IIB fractures with anterior screw fixation, and Type IIC fractures with posterior atlantoaxial spinal fusion.[8]

Despite continued data on the management of fractures of the odontoid process of the axis, the treatment of Type II odontoid fractures remains a source of substantial controversy. Treatment algorithms have evolved over past decades to accommodate differences in fracture pattern as well as patient age, medical condition, and body habitus. Traction and prolonged best rest are now outdated modes of treatment and of historical significance only. Halo vest treatment is also more widely recognized as dangerous in the very elderly population.

Currently, nonsurgical management of Type II fracture involves early immobilization using an alternative external orthosis (e.g., cervical collar, cervicothoracic orthosis). A systematic review of the healing of Type II fractures using these orthoses demonstrated a wide variability, with specific fracture patterns associated with higher rates of healing.[2] Use of traction for 6 weeks followed by a 6-week period of cervical collar immobilization resulted in nonunion in 49% of patients,[2] with a lower rate of nonunion (32%) when more rigid bracing (halo/Minerva cast) was used.[2]

Accepted indications for surgical treatment include a fracture pattern with a high risk of nonunion, proven instability, persistent cord compression in patients with neurologic deficits, and failure of nonsurgical treatment. However, some authors still recommend surgery for all acute Type II fractures, regardless of the risk of nonunion.[9] Surgical strategies include odontoid screw fixation and posterior atlantoaxial arthrodesis. In the case of arthrodesis, autogenous bone graft is most commonly added. The use of allograft and other biologic substitutes has not been adequately studied.

Finally, with an ever-aging world population, surgeons are presented with several challenges when managing odontoid fractures in the elderly, particularly due to the high rate of associated morbidity and mortality. An in-hospital mortality rate of 35% has been observed following odontoid fractures in patients >70 years,[10] and significant care is required when selecting the most appropriate treatment in this age group.[11,12] Several reasons have been postulated for these poorer outcomes, including the mechanism of trauma, poorer rehabilitative potential, the presence of comorbidities, and the consequences of fracture management. The advent of novel surgical techniques in the anterior and posterior upper cervical spine has led to the use of more aggressive fracture management techniques in the older population to facilitate postoperative rehabilitation and avoid rigid bracing.

REFERENCES

1. Hsu WK, Anderson PA. Odontoid fractures: Update on management. *J Am Acad Orthop Surg.* 2010; 18(7): 383–394.
2. Julien TD, Frankel B, Traynelis VC, Ryken TC. Evidence-based analysis of odontoid fracture management. *Neurosurg Focus.* 2000; 8(6): e1.
3. Frangen TM, Zilkens C, Muhr G, Schinkel C. Odontoid fractures in the elderly: Dorsal C1/C2 fusion is superior to halo-vest immobilization. *J Trauma.* 2007; 63(1): 83–89.
4. Müller EJ, Schwinnen I, Fischer K, Wick M, Muhr G. Non-rigid immobilisation of odontoid fractures. *Eur Spine J.* 2003; 12(5): 522–525.
5. Amling M, Hahn M, Wening VJ, Grote HJ, Delling G. The microarchitecture of the axis as the predisposing factor for fracture of the base of the odontoid process: A histomorphometric analysis of twenty-two autopsy specimens. *J Bone Joint Surg Am.* 1994; 76(12): 1840–1846.

6. Clark CR, White AA III. Fractures of the dens: A multicenter study. *J Bone Joint Surg Am*. 1985; 67(9): 1340–1348.
7. Barker L, Anderson J, Chesnut R, Nesbit G, Tjauw T, Hart R. Reliability and reproducibility of dens fracture classification with use of plain radiography and reformatted computer-aided tomography. *J Bone Joint Surg Am*. 2006; 88(1): 106–112.
8. Grauer JN, Shafi B, Hilibrand AS, et al. Proposal of a modified, treatment-oriented classification of odontoid fractures. *Spine J*. 2005; 5(2): 123–129.
9. Apfelbaum RI, Lonser RR, Veres R, Casey A. Direct anterior screw fixation for recent and remote odontoid fractures. *J Neurosurg*. 2000; 93(2 Suppl): 227–236.
10. Müller EJ, Wick M, Russe O, Muhr G. Management of odontoid fractures in the elderly. *Eur Spine J*. 1999; 8(5): 360–365.
11. White AP, Hashimoto R, Norvell DC, Vaccaro AR. Morbidity and mortality related to odontoid fracture surgery in the elderly population. *Spine (Phila Pa 1976)*. 2010; 35(9 Suppl): S146–S157.
12. Butler JS, Dolan RT, Burbridge M, et al. The long-term functional outcome of type II odontoid fractures managed non-operatively. *Eur Spine J*. 2010; 19(10): 1635–1642.

Fractures of the Ring of the Axis: A Classification Based on the Analysis of 131 Cases*

Effendi B, Roy D, Cornish B, Dussault RG, Laurin CA. JBJS 63-B(3):319–327, 1981

Reviewed by Rowan Schouten

Research Question/Objective Prior to 1981, no classification system for fractures of the ring of the axis (C2) existed that delineated the various characteristics of these injuries. This study's primary aim was to produce a radiographic-based classification system that could facilitate treatment decisions and help understand the injury mechanisms involved. Rates of neurological deficits, associated injuries, and mortality rates were documented for each specific fracture type.

Study Design A retrospective analysis of case histories and radiographs.

Sample Size One hundred and thirty-one patients.

Follow-Up Mean 10 months (range 4 months to 4 years).

Inclusion/Extrusion Criteria All patients had a fracture of the ring of the axis (C2), defined as involving the lamina, articular facets, pars, pedicles, or the posterior wall of the C2 vertebra. Their injuries were managed at centers in Canada and Australia. Each had a minimum 4-month follow-up and had available complete clinical notes together with original and final radiographs. The available imaging studies varied but included static and dynamic (flexion/extension) plain X-rays, supplemented by tomograms, and computerized axial tomography (CAT) scans.

Intervention The treatment of each fracture was retrospectively documented. Options utilized included bracing, halo-thoracic

---

* Effendi B, Roy D, Cornish B, Dussault RG, Laurin CA. Fractures of the ring of the axis: A classification based on the analysis of 131 cases. *J Bone Joint Surg Br.* 1981; 63-B(3): 319–327.

immobilization, traction, open reduction, and posterior C2-C3 interspinous wiring or anterior C2-C3 fusion.

Results   All fractures were classified into 3 types based on the degree of fracture displacement coupled with the status of the C2-C3 disc and facet joints (Figure 13.1).

Type I injuries involved isolated *hairline* (<1 mm) fractures with minimum displacement of the C2 body and an intact C2-C3 disc space. Type II injuries involved displacement (>1 mm) of the C2 body with a disrupted C2-C3 disc. In Type III injuries, the C2 body was displaced and the C2-C3 disc space was disrupted with concomitant dislocation of the C2-C3 facets.

The authors recommended that injuries without initial displacement or obvious disruption of the C2-C3 disc should undergo lateral flexion/extension radiographs "taken without anesthesia, while an experienced clinician exerts mild manual traction." Injuries stable on these dynamic images were classified as Type I.

Within the study cohort, the incidence of each fracture type was 65%, 28%, and 7% for Type I, II, and III injuries, respectively. Overall, the mean age was 31 years, 73% were males, and 72% resulted from motor vehicle accidents. Fourteen percent had associated cervical spine injuries. Nine (7%) patients died; however, in only 3 deaths was the axis fracture considered responsible, the others succumbing to associated injuries.

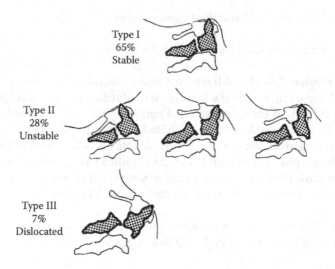

Type I
65%
Stable

Type II
28%
Unstable

Type III
7%
Dislocated

Figure 13.1   Fracture types and incidence from the original article outlining the classification system proposed by Effendi et al. (Reproduced with permission and copyright © of the British Editorial Society of Bone and Joint Surgery: Effendi, B. et al., *J. Bone Joint Surg. Br.*, 63-B(3), 319–327, 1984.)

Permanent neurological deficits resulting from fractures of the axis were uncommon. In all patients with Type I fractures, no permanent neurological deficits were directly attributed to the axis injury, while only one of 37 cases of Type II injuries and one of the 9 Type III injuries sustained permanent neurological deficits. Severe neurological deficits were more commonly the result of noncontiguous spinal cord trauma or vertebral artery insufficiency.

For Type I injuries, 6 weeks in a brace was recommended. Type II lesions were considered best managed in a halo-thoracic vest for 12 weeks, which could be preceded by up to 3 weeks of skull traction to realign and reduce any displacement between the C2 and C3 vertebrae. For Type II injuries, the authors state "there is no place for an immediate fusion," and only if instability is noted on flexion/extension films following 12 weeks of immobilization is an anterior fusion of C2 and C3 *justified*. For Type III injuries, open reduction of the dislocated facets with interspinous wiring of C2 to C3, effectively converting this injury to an equivalent Type II injury, with management in a halo-thoracic vest for 12 weeks was advocated.

The proposed injury mechanism was forceful hyperextension and axial loading for type I and II injuries. Type III injuries were considered to result from forceful flexion initially, to create the C2-C3 facet joint dislocation, followed by rebound extension and axial loading to cause the axis fracture.

Study Limitations With limited number of fractures included in the cohort, the potential exists that a specific fracture pattern that occurs only rarely may be overlooked. The study's retrospective nature also meant patients often received more surgical intervention than the final proposed treatment regime recommended. Prospective outcome studies are therefore required before this treatment algorithm can be validated.

The role of advanced imaging modalities has significantly expanded since this study. In contrast to the authors comment that "CAT scans are rarely necessary," multiplanar reformatted CT scanning provides detailed imaging of the fracture anatomy and is now regarded by many as the preferred primary screening modality in cervical trauma.[1] The author's preference for dynamic radiographs obtained with the application of manual traction in the acute trauma setting is now rarely justified. Magnetic resonance imaging (MRI) provides a more contemporary method of assessing occult injury to the C2-C3 disc and associated soft tissues.

Relevant Studies Despite multiple aliases, including *Hangman's fractures* and *traumatic spondylolisthesis of the axis*, few attempts at classifying this group of injuries exist. Earlier attempts and the simultaneous 1981 classification system of Francis et al.,[2] based on White and Panjabi's limits of 3.5 mm of displacement and 11 degrees of angulation, have been largely discarded.

Levine and Edwards[3] modified the original Effendi et al. classification in 1985 to create a system of four C2 ring fracture types (Type I, II, IIa, III) that remains the most widely used. They proposed that each injury type resulted from a specific mechanism that then formed the basis for their treatment decisions. Type I fractures had less than 3 mm of displacement and no angulation. While the degree of displacement differed from that proposed by Effendi et al. (<1 mm), the predicted mechanism involving pure hyperextension with axial loading and the recommended treatment in a cervical collar was identical. Type II injuries showed significant angulation and translation (>3 mm). In contrast to the Type II injuries identified by Effendi et al., Levine and Edwards noted a subset of fractures (designated Type IIa) with slight or no translation but severe angulation. When halo traction was applied to these patients, immediate widening of the posterior C2-C3 disc space was noted. They postulated that the common Type II fractures resulted from combination hyperextension–axial loading with secondary flexion-compression. In contrast, the Type IIa injuries were caused by flexion-distraction, which formed the basis for the recommended treatment option involving application of mild compression-extension in a halo vest under fluoroscopic guidance. The characteristics of Type III injuries were not changed, but in contrast to Effendi et al., they considered Type III injuries to have resulted from flexion-compression. For this cohort, surgical reduction and stabilization was again indicated.

Fractures of the ring of the axis are typically associated with low rates of neurological injury[3] as displacement of most fracture patterns results in spinal canal expansion. However, Starr et al. in 1993 highlighted that fractures involving the posterior cortex of C2, when accompanied by translation, can result in canal compression causing neurological dysfunction (Figure 13.2). They suggested

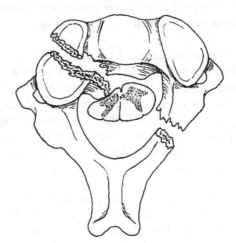

Figure 13.2 Schematic drawing showing spinal cord compression from anterior displacement of an atypical Hangman's fracture. (Reprinted with permission from Starr, J.K. and Eismont, F.J., *Spine (Phila Pa 1976)*, 18, 1954–1957, 1993.)

these *atypical Hangman fractures* should be recognized as distinct injuries that require greater vigilance.[4]

The classification system proposed by Effendi et al. and modified by Levine and Edwards continues to provide the framework for ongoing debate about management of these injuries. While broad consistency exists for the treatment of Type I injuries, currently there remains no consensus on the optimal treatment of Type II, IIa, and III fractures. Since the publication of Effendi et al., surgical stabilization via anterior C2-C3 fusion or posterior approaches has become more commonplace. This trend has been spurred on by the advent of modern cervical spine instrumentation and assisted by technology such as surgical navigation systems that permit safe and accurate placement of posterior cervical screws.[5] Results of a 2010 questionnaire of 77 spinal trauma surgeons across four continents showed surgical stabilization was the preferred treatment option for Type II injuries among European and Asian surgeons, while North American and Australasian surgeons favored halo-thoracic brace therapy.[6]

REFERENCES

1. Como JJ, Diaz JJ, Dunham CM, et al. Practice management guidelines for identification of cervical spine injuries following trauma: Update from the Eastern Association for the Surgery of Trauma practice management guidelines committee. *J Trauma*. 2009; 67(3): 651–659.
2. Francis WR, Fielding JW, Hawkins RJ, Pepin J, Hensinger R. Traumatic spondylolisthesis of the axis. *J Bone Joint Surg Br*. 1981; 63-B(3): 313–318.
3. Levine AM, Edwards CC. The management of traumatic spondylolisthesis of the axis. *J Bone Joint Surg*. 1985; 67(2): 217–226.
4. Starr JK, Eismont FJ. Atypical hangman's fractures. *Spine*. 1993; 18(14): 1954–1957.
5. Singh PK, Garg K, Sawarkar D, et al. Computed tomography-guided C2 pedicle screw placement for treatment of unstable hangman fractures. *Spine*. 2014; 39(18): E1058–E1065.
6. Lenehan B, Dvorak MF, Madrazo I, Yukawa Y, Fisher CG. Diversity and commonalities in the care of spine trauma internationally. *Spine*. 2010; 35(21 Suppl): S174–S179.

CHAPTER 14

A New Classification of Thoracolumbar Injuries: The Importance of Injury Morphology, the Integrity of the Posterior Ligamentous Complex, and Neurological Status*

Vaccaro AR, Lehman RA, Hurlbert R. John, et al. Spine 30:2325–2333, 2005

Reviewed by Jefferson R. Wilson and Alex Vaccaro

Research Question/Objective   Fractures involving the thoracolumbar spine are common, necessitating a simple and reliable method by which such injuries can be systematically characterized in order to facilitate communication, diagnosis, and treatment. Previous classifications were felt to be overly complex, dismissive of anatomical features that affect treatment decision making, and not practically useful in helping surgeons decide on the suitability of operative versus nonoperative treatment. The central goal of the current study was to devise a new thoracolumbar classification to overcome the aforementioned limitations of previous systems.

Study Design   A literature review of previous thoracolumbar classification systems was completed. Subsequent to the review, a two-part survey of members of the Spine Trauma Study Group (STSG) was completed, first, to achieve consensus regarding the principle categories to be included in the classification and, second, to identify pitfalls and opportunities for improvement.

Sample Size   Forty surgical spine experts from 15 level 1 trauma institutions in 9 countries were involved in forming the expert STSG panel that participated in classification development.

Follow-Up   Not applicable.

---

* Vaccaro AR, Lehman RA, Hurlbert RJ, et al. A new classification of thoracolumbar injuries: The importance of injury morphology, the integrity of the posterior ligamentous complex, and neurological status. *Spine*. 2005; 30: 2325–2333.

Inclusion/Exclusion Criteria   Eligibility criteria for studies included in the review of literature were not articulated within the manuscript.

Intervention   Not applicable.

Results   A classification with three main variables was identified: Injury Morphology, Integrity of Posterior Ligamentous Complex (PLC), and Neurological Status (Table 14.1). Within each of these categories, subcategories were identified and assigned a point system so that a higher overall point score represents a greater injury severity as well as perceived need for operative intervention. Within the category of injury morphology, subcategories, in order of ascending severity, included compression morphology (1 point or 2 points with the burst fracture modifier), distraction morphology (3 points), and translation morphology (4 points). For the category of PLC integrity, subcategories included intact (0 points), suspected/indeterminate (2 points), injured (3 points). Disruption of PLC is indicated by splaying of the spinous processes, diastasis of facet joints, and facet perch or subluxation. When disruption is suspected but not obvious, such as the situation of ligamentous hyperintensity on T2 STIR MRI with no definitive splaying or diastasis seen, PLC injury is categorized as suspect/indeterminate. Finally, for neurological status, subcategories included intact (0 points), single root injury (2 points), complete spinal cord or conus injury (2 points), incomplete spinal cord or conus injury (3 points), and cauda equina injury (3 points). The increased number of points allocated to incomplete cord/conus injuries and cauda equina injuries, compared to incomplete injuries, was indicative of consensus among STSG members that the former represent a greater degree of

Table 14.1   Thoracolumbar Injury Severity Score (TLICS)

Injury Severity Score: Thoracolumbar Injury Classification and Severity Score (TLICS)	1. Pattern or morphology: Comparable to type level of AO system
	a. Compression = 1 point
	b. Burst = 2 points
	c. Rotation/translation = 3 points
	d. Distraction = 4 points
	2. Posterior ligamentary complex integrity: Working as a tension band
	a. Intact = 0 point
	b. Suspected/intermediate = 2 points
	c. Disrupted = 3 points
	3. Neurologic involvement: One of the most crucial parameters in clinical decision making
	a. Intact = 0 point
	b. Nerve root = 2 points
	c. Cord/conus
	d. Complete (ASIA A) = 2 points
	e. Incomplete (ASIA B-D) = 3 points
	f. Cauda equina = 3 points

Table 14.2   Suggested Treatment Decision Making Based on Score from SLIC and TLICS

Score interpretation	Sum of scores yields severity score:
	• ≤3 points = nonoperative
	• ≥5 points = operative
	• 4 points = nonoperative or operative

surgical urgency given their perceived potential for enhanced recovery with surgical intervention compared to those with complete injuries.

The point system was designed so that summating points across each of the three categories for a given injury results in a comprehensive severity score, which can be then used to determine individuals' operative candidacy (Table 14.2); a comprehensive severity score of 3 or less suggests a nonoperative injury, while a score of 5 or more suggests that surgical intervention may be considered. Injuries with a score of 4 might be handled conservatively or surgically. In addition to the comprehensive severity score, the authors suggest a series of patient-specific modifiers including local factors such as extreme kyphosis; multiple rib fractures or open fractures; as well as systemic considerations, in turn including the rheumatoid arthritis, ankylosing spondylitis, or advanced age, which might affect operative decision making.

Study Limitations   In this particular study, the psychometrics of the classification system are not directly reported. Therefore, important information surrounding its reliability and validity was not made available here. Second, while this system provides direction regarding whether operative or nonoperative treatment should be pursued for a given patient, the system itself provides little direction with respect to the type of operation that should be performed (i.e., anterior versus posterior versus combined, number of fusion levels, etc.). Third, while integrity of the PLC is an extremely important consideration when conceptualizing spinal stability, there is a paucity of practical information included within this article to guide clinicians on how best to assess the PLC using clinical exam and imaging. Finally, although the modifiers are important to ensure patient-specific considerations are incorporated when making treatment decisions, it is somewhat unclear how the authors expect these to be used, in combination with the comprehensive severity score, to decide on individuals' operative candidacy.

Relevant Studies   The principal forerunners to the Thoracolumbar Injury Classification System (TLICS) classification were the Denis[1,2] and the Magerl (AO)[3] classification systems. While these are recognized as valuable tools that have advanced our ability to categorize and understand spine trauma, each has significant drawbacks. Specifically, the Magerl classification, in its attempt to provide a comprehensive catalog of injury patterns, is quite complex and cumbersome to apply in the real world. Not unsurprising, interobserver reliability was found to be only fair (kappa = 0.34) with this classification. While the Denis three-column classification system is more practical for use and reliable (kappa = 0.60), the interpretation that injury involvement of two contiguous columns results in mechanical instability is contraindicated by the fact that nonoperative treatment of burst fractures, which compromise the anterior and middle column, is successful in many cases. In addition to the above, neither classification includes assessment of neurological status in determining injury severity, nor does either provide a specific algorithm to decide on whether operative or nonoperative treatment is most suitable for a given injury. On these grounds, TLICS ostensibly represents a major advancement over previous systems designed to categorize thoracolumbar spinal trauma.

Although not addressed specifically in the primary article, additional follow-up studies have shown TLICS to be valid and reliable, with moderate to substantial interrater reliability (kappa values 0.45–0.74) and substantial intrarater reliability (kappa = 0.73).[4,5] Such reliability has been documented for both neurosurgeons and orthopedic surgeons alike in numerous practice settings internationally.[6] With respect to individual categories, integrity of the posterior ligamentous complex has shown in multiple studies to demonstrate the poorest reliability statistics, with a kappa statistic ranging from as low as 0.29 is one study to as high as 0.72 in a follow-up study.[4–6] More recently, TLICS has also been shown to be valid and reliable in the pediatric spine trauma population.[7]

After publication of the primary article, for purposes of knowledge translation, a number of follow-up articles were published by members of the STSG to provide clear instruction and practical illustration of how TLICS can be applied by surgeons to commonly encountered thoracolumbar trauma cases.[8]

REFERENCES

1. Denis F. The three-column spine and its significance in the classification of thoracolumbar spinal injuries. *Spine*. 1983; 817–831.
2. McAfee PC, Yuan HA, Fredrickson BE, et al. The value of computed tomography in thoracolumbar fractures: An analysis of one hundred consecutive cases and a new classification. *J Bone Jt Surg, Am Volume*. 1983; 65: 461–473.
3. Magerl F, Aebi M, Gertzbein SD, et al. A comprehensive classification of thoracic and lumbar injuries. *Eur Spine J*. 1994; 3: 184–201.
4. Lewkonia P, Oddone Paolucci E, Thomas K. Reliability of the Thoracolumbar Injury Classification and Severity Score and comparison with the Denis classification for injury to thoracic and lumbar spine. *Spine*. 2012; 26: 2151–2167.
5. Whang PG, Vaccaro AR, Poelstra KA, et al. The influence of fracture mechanism and morphology on the reliability and validity of two novel thoracolumbar injury classification systems. *Spine*. 2007; 32: 791.

6. Rampersaud R, Fisher C, Wilsey J, et al. Agreement between orthopedic surgeons and neurosurgeons regarding a new algorithm for the treatment of thoracolumbar injuries: A multicenter reliability study. *J Spinal Disord Techniq*. 2006; 19: 477.

7. Savage JW, Moore TA, Arnold PM, et al. The reliability and validity of the Thoracolumbar Injury Classification System in Pediatric Spine Trauma. *Spine*. 2015; 40: E1014–E1018.

8. Patel AA, Dailey A, Brodke DS, et al. Thoracolumbar spine trauma classification: The Thoracolumbar Injury Classification and Severity Score system and case examples. *J Neurosurg Spine*. 2009; 10: 201–206.

CHAPTER 15

A Comprehensive Classification of Thoracic and Lumbar Injuries*

Magerl F, Aebi M, Gertzbein SD, et al. Eur Spine J 3:184–201, 1994

Reviewed by Elsa Arocho-Quiñones, Hesham Soliman, and Shekar Kurpad

Research Question/Objective   Nearly 50% of all spine fractures involve the thoracic and lumbar spine.[1] Given the frequency of thoracic and lumbar fractures and the numerous treatment options, there is a need for a comprehensive classification system to enhance communication, and facilitate diagnosis and treatment selection. Such a classification system would allow the identification of any injury by means of a simple algorithm based on radiographic and clinical characteristics, ultimately leading to a concise stratification of the mechanism of injury as well as the injury severity, which would in turn help guide the choice of treatment.

Previous studies and proposed classification systems were not considered all-inclusive. The goal of this study was to devise a classification system for thoracic and lumbar injuries that would meet the aforementioned criteria.

Study Design   A literature review of previous classification systems for thoracic and lumbar injuries was completed. This was followed by a thorough review of 1445 consecutive thoracolumbar injuries at five institutions.† Several existing classification systems were tested and a new classification system was developed.

The 1445 cases investigated were analyzed with regard to (1) the level of the main injury, (2) the frequency of the different types and groups of injuries, and (3) the incidence of neurological deficit.

Sample Size   A total of 1445 consecutive thoracolumbar injuries at five institutions were reviewed.

* Magerl F, Aebi M, Gertzbein SD, et al. A comprehensive classification of thoracic and lumbar injuries. *Eur Spine J.* 1994; 3: 184–201.

† Department of Orthopaedic Surgery, Kantonsspital, St. Gallen; Department of Orthopaedic Surgery, Inselspital, Bern; Sunnybrook Health Service Centre, Toronto; Rehabilitationskrankenhaus, Karlsbad-Langensteinbach; Hospital de la Conception, Marseille, France.

Follow-Up   Not applicable.

Inclusion/Exclusion Criteria   Isolated transverse or spinous process fractures were not considered in the classification.

Intervention or Treatment Received   Not applicable.

Results   This proposed classification system is based primarily on the pathomorphology of the injury, with particular emphasis on the extent of involvement of the anterior and posterior elements. The 3-3-3 scheme of the AO fracture classification was used in grouping the injuries.[2] There are three main types of injuries, and every type in turn has three groups, each of which contains three subgroups with specifications. The three principal types are determined by the three key mechanisms acting on the spine: compression (A), distraction (B), and torsion (C).[3] Predominantly morphological criteria were used for all further grouping.

The severity of trauma was considered in the organization of the classification and progressed from Type A through Type C as well as within the types, groups, and subgroups. The severity of the injury was defined by the presence of instability, risk of neurologic injury, and prognostic aspects for healing. The loss of stability constituted the primary determining factor for ranking the injuries because it is the most important factor for choosing the form of treatment.

Most injuries were primarily located around the thoracolumbar junction. The levels least affected included the upper and lower ends of the thoracolumbar spine as well as the T10 level.

Type A fractures represented two-thirds of all injuries, with Type B and C lesions accounting for the remaining one-third of injuries. A more detailed analysis performed on 468 of the 1445 cases revealed that 23% had multisegmental injuries within the thoracolumbar spine. The frequency of Type A injuries decreased in a cranial to caudal fashion, whereas Type B injuries occurred more often around the thoracolumbar junction, and Type C injuries were more frequently located in the lumbar spine.

The incidence of neurological deficit (ranging from single root injury to complete paraplegia) was evaluated in 1212 of 1445 patients. The overall incidence of neurological deficit was 22%. The incidence of neurological deficit within types was 14% for Type A injuries, 35% for Type B injuries, and 55% for Type C injuries, thus indicating that the risk of neurological injury is related to the degree of instability. The authors also incorporated prognostic aspects into the organization of the proposed classification system and made a distinction between purely osseous injuries and discoligamentous injuries, since the latter injuries increase instability and have poor healing potential.[4] The degree of instability and the risk of neurological injury is therefore reflected by ranking within this classification and increases from type to type and within each subdivision.

General recommendations regarding treatment were as follows: Type A injuries ranged from the stable A1 fractures to the very unstable A3.3 burst fractures. Because the tensile strength is unimpaired when the anterior longitudinal ligament (ALL) is preserved and the posterior elements maintain their stabilizing function as long as the posterior longitudinal ligaments (PLLs) are preserved, conservative or nonoperative treatment is possible when the ALL and PLL are preserved. In Type B1 and B2 injuries, the stability in flexion is almost always completely lost due to the transverse posterior disruption. Type B injuries may also have partial or complete loss of tensile strength if associated with a Type A fracture. The treatment of these injuries should involve posterior compression and restoration of the compressive resistance of the anterior column, which may be accomplished conservatively for mostly osseous injuries with intact articular processes, whereas mostly discoligamentous injuries necessitate surgical treatment and fusion. All Type B3 injuries have disc disruption and therefore require surgical treatment with fusion. Anterior fusion followed by postoperative immobilization may be applied to injuries with preserved stability in flexion, whereas posterior dislocations and some shear fracture dislocations require anterior and posterior stabilization. Type C injuries are unstable in axial torque and may be combined with Type A or B injuries. These injuries often include avulsion of soft tissue attachments, including discoligamentous structures and fractures of bony structures responsible for rotational resistance (e.g., transverse processes, ribs). Type C injuries are considered the most unstable and had the highest incidence of neurological injury (55%); as such, these rotational injuries require surgical stabilization with the aim of stabilizing axial torque and shearing in the horizontal plane in addition to resisting flexion/extension forces associated with Type A and Type B fractures occurring in combination or separately.

Study Limitations   Although this classification system offers a comprehensive way to describe and stratify the various injury patterns affecting the thoracolumbar spine by spine surgeons, it is complex, with consequent limitation in practical application. The proper classification of these injury patterns relies on thorough and expert analysis of imaging studies and is therefore dependent on evaluator expertise and subject to interobserver variability; validation mechanisms for such variability is not provided in the primary article. In the article, specific imaging modalities that assisted in generating the classification are somewhat unclear (plain films versus CT), resulting in erroneous assignment to Type A injuries (when the correct diagnosis with more advanced imaging might have assigned these to Type B injuries). Finally, while the study was intended to furnish a classification paradigm that would assist in the selection of appropriate treatment, a specific algorithm for such selection was not described in this study.

Relevant Studies   Several studies leading to the development of previous classification systems were instrumental in adding to the knowledge and understanding of spinal injuries. For instance, Whitesides et al. recognized a mechanistic classification and defined the two-column concept.[3] Louis et al. used a morphological classification system instituting the concept of three columns (consisting of vertebral bodies and two rows of the articular masses) and differentiated between transient osseous instability and chronic instability secondary to discoligamentous injuries.[4] Studies by Denis et al. led to the development of the three-column classification, where the anterior column is composed of the anterior longitudinal ligament, the anterior annulus, and the anterior aspect of the vertebral body; the middle column is composed of the posterior longitudinal ligament, the posterior annulus, and the posterior aspect of the vertebral body; and the posterior column includes the neural arch, facet joints, ligamentum flavum, and interspinous ligament complex. In the Denis classification, "the third column represented the structures that would need to be torn in addition to the posterior ligament complex in order to create acute instability."[5–7] These previous systems, however, were not comprehensive as they did not include assessment of neurological status in the determination of injury severity, nor did they offer an algorithm for the selection of treatment options. A more recently proposed classification system by Vaccaro et al. represents an improvement over previous classification schemes as it is based on injury morphology, integrity of the posterior ligamentous complex, and neurological status. This classification scheme offers a point-based system, where a higher overall point score represents a greater injury severity and perceived need for surgical intervention proven to be valid and reliable in several studies.[8–10]

REFERENCES

1. Ghobrial GM, Senders ZJ, Harrop JS. (2016, February 22). *Vertebral Fracture*. Retrieved December 04, 2017, from https://emedicine.medscape.com/article/248236-overview#a5.
2. Muller ME, Nazarian S, Koch P (1987) Classification AO des fractures. 1 Les os longs. Springer, Berlin Heidelberg New York.
3. Whitesides TE Jr. Traumatic kyphosis of the thoracolumbar spine. *Clin Orthop Relat Res*. 1977; 128: 78–92.
4. Louis R. Les theories de l'instabilite. *Rev Chir Orthop*. 1977; 63: 423–425.
5. Denis F. Updated classification of thoracolumbar fractures. *Orthop Trans*. 1982; 6: 8–9.
6. Denis F. The three-column spine and its significance in the classification of acute thoraco-lumbar spinal injuries. *Spine*. 1983; 8: 817–831.
7. Denis F. Spinal instability as defined by the three-column spine concept in acute spinal trauma. *Clin Orthop*. 1984; 189: 65–76.
8. Vaccaro AR, Lehman RA, Hurlbert J, et al. A new classification of thoracolumbar injuries: The importance of injury morphology, the integrity of the posterior ligamentous complex, and neurological status. *Spine*. 2005; 30: 2325–2333.

9. Lewkonia P, Oddone Paolucci E, Thomas K. Reliability of the Thoracolumbar Injury Classification and Severity Score and Comparison with the Denis Classification for Injury to Thoracic and Lumbar Spine. *Spine*. 2012; 26: 2151–2167.
10. Whang PG, Vaccaro AR, Poelstra KA, et al. The influence of fracture mechanism and morphology on the reliability and validity of two novel thoracolumbar injury classification systems. *Spine*. 2007; 32: 791.

CHAPTER 16

International Standards for Neurological Classification of Spinal Cord Injury (ISNCSCI)*

Kirshblum SC, Burns SP, Biering-Sorensen F, Donovan W, Graves DE, Jha A, Johansen M, Jones L, Krassioukov A, Mulcahey MJ, Schmidt-Read M, Waring W. 34(6):535–546, 2011

Reviewed by Sukhvinder Kalsi-Ryan

Research Question/Objective   The objective of this paper is to present the 2011 version of the international standards for neurological classification of spinal cord injury, specifically the new instruction booklet, which presents the new and revised methodology to administer the exam along with the revised rules for classification.

Study Design   This manuscript presents the proceedings of the ASIA Standards Committee and the final results of the work done to revise the ISNCSCI in 2011. Currently the 2011 version of the ISNCSCI is the most current version of the test protocol. There have been two revisions to the score sheet since 2011, one in 2013 and 2015. The most current version of the scoring sheet is the 2015 version.

Sample Size   Not applicable.

Follow-Up   Not applicable.

Inclusion/Exclusion Criteria   Not applicable.

Intervention or Treatment Received   Not applicable.

Results   New version of the ISNCSCI and a revised booklet.

Study Limitations   Not applicable.

---

* Kirshblum SC, Burns SP, Biering-Sorensen F, et al. International standards for neurological classification of spinal cord injury (revised 2011). *J Spinal Cord Med.* 2011; 34(6): 535–546.

Relevant Studies   The latest revision of the International Standards for the Neurological Classification of Spinal Cord Injury (ISNCSCI) was made available in booklet format in June 2011, and subsequently published in this manuscript. The ISNCSCI was initially developed in 1982 to provide standardization for classification of neurological level and extent of spinal cord injury (SCI) to achieve consistent data for clinical care and research studies. The 2011 revision was generated from the Standards Committee of the American Spinal Injury Association in collaboration with the International Spinal Cord Society's Education Committee.

A companion paper was also published in the same issue of *Journal of Spinal Cord Medicine* titled "Reference for the 2011 Revision of the International Standards for Neurological Classification of Spinal Cord Injury."[1] This article details and explains the updates and serves as a reference for the revisions and clarifications presented in the manuscript under review. The original ASIA Standards developed in 1982 defined neurological levels and the extent of the injury utilizing the Frankel Scale[2,3] to achieve greater consistency and reliable data among centers participating in the National SCI Statistical Center Database. Subsequently, major revisions have been made in 1990, 1992, 1996, and 2000.[4] In 1992, the International Spinal Cord Society (ISCoS), endorsed the standards, and at that time the standards were renamed the International Standards for Neurological Classification of Spinal Cord Injury (ISNCSCI).[5]

The first reference manual was published in 1994, with an updated version in 2003.[6,7] In 2010, the International Standards Training e-Learning Program (InSTeP) was developed by ASIA, which incorporated the updated recommendations for the neurological examination and classification; this excellent learning tool has been available online since 2010.[8] The InSTeP includes a six-module course, which educates clinicians about how to perform the exam accurately and consistently. The modules included in the InSTeP are Basic Anatomy; Sensory Examination; Motor Examination; Anorectal Examination; Scoring, Scaling, and the ASIA Impairment Scale (AIS) Classification; and Optional Testing. The purpose of the ISNCSCI is to facilitate accurate and consistent assessment for communication among clinicians and researchers working with spinal-cord-injured patients; the purpose remains unchanged from the original intent 25 years ago.

Despite the consistent use and implementation of the standards since the inception of the tool, there have been many challenges with the development process. The ISNCSCI did go through an arduous item generation and reduction process, which confirmed the content of the tool. However, there has been little done to establish the sensibility and psychometric properties. There are a few reliability studies in adults, and prior to 2008, three studies did indicate that the interrater reliability was too low to consider the ISNCSCI as an outcome measure for clinical trials.[9,10] However, in 2008 an interrater reliability study did confirm that reliability could be above 0.80 (intra-class correlation coefficient) if a standardized training is provided prior to testing.[11] Another challenge in using ISNCSCI scores was related to large total scores that represented the whole body rather than specific segments. Sensitivity of the ISNCSCI was enhanced when it was confirmed that the upper extremity motor scores (UEMSs) and lower extremity motor scores (LEMSs) could be used as separate scores. Use of the UEMS for tetraplegia and LEMS for paraplegia has become common practice, which provides more resolution regarding the patient's impairment than motor levels.

The ISNCSCI was developed as a classification tool to define spinal cord function based on assessment at the periphery. The concept has been designed to document the most caudal level at which the spinal cord has normal function in a noninvasive manner. However, the research field has adopted the ISNCSCI as a primary outcome measure in many studies and, as a result, have found the tool not to be adequate for this purpose. The ISNCSCI was never designed to be a primary outcome measure; it was meant to be a classification tool. Nonetheless, these criticisms have led the developers to continue revising the measure over the years, resulting in a useful classification measure that is now considered a *gold standard*. It is important for clinicians who use this tool to truly understand the meaning of the processed scores. Assigning neurological levels and the ASIA Impairment Scale (AIS) rating can be confusing if there is not a thorough understanding of how to assign the raw scores.

Currently, the ISNCSCI is considered a *gold standard* measure in the management of traumatic SCI. With the 2011 revision, administration of the ISNCSCI has become much more standardized than previous versions. Still the field should continue to consider how this assessment tool should be used. Furthermore, a true understanding by clinicians in the output of the measure is mandatory for use of the tool to be appropriate. This can only be done with ongoing education and instruction regarding the purpose of the tool, how it is administered, how a score and classification is derived, and what the output actually represents in relation to spinal cord function.

Moving forward, the ASIA International Standards Committee has adopted a review process and, if needed, will revise the ISNCSCI every 3 years. It is necessary not only to teach how to accurately administer ISNCSCI (which the committee has done well with the dissemination of the 2011 revisions and the InSTep) but also to ensure that assessors understand what the scores actually mean. This can be done through historical datasets, which can inform the field of what temporal score changes represent in the recovery process of traumatic SCI. In summary, the 2011 version of the ISNCSCI has resolved many of the challenges faced by the field with respect to standardization. The primary emphasis at this stage is to ensure the appropriate, accurate use and understanding of the tool and meaning of scores.

REFERENCES

1. Kirshblum S, Waring W, Biering-Sorensen F, et al. Reference for the 2011 revision of the International Standards for Neurological Classification of Spinal Cord Injury. *JSCM*. 2011; 34(6): 457–454.
2. Frankel HL, Hancock DO, Hyslop G, et al. The value of postural reduction in the initial management of closed injuries in the spine with paraplegia and tetraplegia. *Paraplegia*. 1969; 7: 179–192.
3. American Spinal Injury Association. *Standards for Neurological Classification of Spinal Injured Patients*. Chicago, IL: ASIA; 1982.
4. American Spinal Injury Association. *International Standards for Neurological Classification of Spinal cord Injury*. Atlanta, GA; revised 2000; reprinted 2008.
5. American Spinal Injury Association/International Medical Society of Paraplegia (ASIA/IMSOP). *International Standards for Neurological and Functional Classification of Spinal Cord Injury Patients (Revised)*. Chicago, IL: American Spinal Injury Association; 1996.
6. Marino RJ, Barros T, Biering-Sorensen F, et al. International standards for neurological classification of spinal cord injury. *JSCM*. 2003; 26(Suppl 1): S50–S56.
7. American Spinal Injury Association. *Reference Manual for the International Standards for Neurological Classification of Spinal Cord Injury*. Chicago, IL: American Spinal Injury Association; 2003.
8. American Spinal Injury Association ASIA Learning Center. [accessed 2011 Oct 5]. Available from www.asialearningcenter.com.
9. Jonsson M, Tollbäck A, Gonzales H, Borg J. Inter-rater reliability of the 1992 international standards for neurological and functional classification of incomplete spinal cord injury. *Spinal Cord*. 2000; 38(11): 675–679.
10. Mulcahey MJ, Gaughan J, Betz RR, Vogel LC. Rater agreement on the ISCSCI motor and sensory scores obtained before and after formal training in testing technique. *JSCM*. 2007; 30(Suppl 1): S146–S149.
11. Marino RJ, Jones L, Kirshblum S, Tal J, Dasgupta A. Reliability and repeatability of the motor and sensory examination of the international standards for neurological classification of spinal cord injury. *JSCM*. 2008; 31(2): 166–170.

New Technologies in Spine: Kyphoplasty and Vertebroplasty for the Treatment of Painful Osteoporotic Compression Fractures*

Garfin SR, Yuan HA, Reiley MA. Spine 26(14):1511–1515, 2001

Reviewed by Clifford Lin

Research Question/Objective   To describe new treatments for painful osteoporotic compression fractures in light of available scientific literature and clinical experience.

Study Design   Literature review.

Sample Size   Not applicable.

Follow-Up   Not applicable.

Inclusion/Exclusion Criteria   Eligibility criteria for studies included in the review of literature were not articulated within the manuscript.

Intervention   Not applicable.

Results   Osteoporotic vertebral compression fractures have a significant negative impact on quality of life, physical function, mental health, and mortality.[†] This study reviewed the literature surrounding the vertebral augmentation procedures vertebroplasty and kyphoplasty as treatments for vertebral compression fractures. It found generally favorable results with a reported success rate in pain relief of 70%–90%. Most patients also had decreased narcotic requirements following these procedures. Additionally, patients who underwent kyphoplasty had some reduction in

---

* Garfin SR, et al. New technologies in spine: Kyphoplasty and vertebroplasty for the treatment of painful osteoporotic compression fractures. *Spine*. 2001; 26(14): 1511–1515.
† Ibid.

their deformity. The average anterior height was 83% ± 14% pretreatment and 99% ± 13% posttreatment ($p < 0.01$). In cases where vertebral height loss was greater than 15 degrees, the average anterior height was 68% ± 12% pretreatment and 84% ± 14% following treatment ($p < 0.01$).

Overall reported complication rate for both procedures was low (less than 10%). With vertebroplasty, cement leakage occurred with an incidence of 30%–67%; however, this did not generally lead to clinically significant sequelae. Radiculopathy occurred at a rate of 4%, and cord compression occurred at a rate of less than 0.5%. The majority of reported symptoms were transient. With kyphoplasty, four important complications were reported: transient fever and hypoxia as a result of PMMA injection, epidural hematoma, delivery of cement into the spinal canal, and a case of anterior cord syndrome as a complication of needle insertion. However, complications were still rare, with an overall reported rate of 0.7% per fracture and 1.2% per patient.

The authors of this study assert that vertebral augmentation procedures (VAPs) are an effective means of rapid pain relief and return to function with a low rate of major complications.

Study Limitations   The authors provide a comprehensive summary of the data available to them at the time. However, much of the literature reviewed in this article is Level 3 or 4 evidence based on uncontrolled prospective studies or case studies, which weakens the strength of their conclusions. Additional Level 1 data has been published subsequent to this article, which casts a different light on the use of vertebral augmentation procedures. These contemporary studies will be discussed below.

Relevant Studies   This study by Garfin et al. was published in 2001, and at the time, vertebral augmentation procedures were enjoying great success, supported by a large body of evidence, albeit of low quality. The first randomized controlled trial comparing kyphoplasty to nonsurgical care reported that kyphoplasty resulted in superior primary and secondary outcomes up to 12 months, after which the groups had similar outcomes.[1] This study was criticized for not being blinded. Klazen et al., in another open-label randomized trial comparing vertebroplasty to conservative treatment, demonstrated improved pain and function scores with vertebroplasty over 12 months follow-up.[2] Contrary to these studies, the *New England Journal of Medicine* (*NEJM*) published two landmark studies by Buchbinder et al. and Kallmes et al. in 2009, which had a significant impact on the practice of VAPs.[3,4] These were prospective, randomized, double-blinded, placebo-controlled studies comparing vertebroplasty to a sham procedure in patients with osteoporotic vertebral compression fractures. These studies did not show any difference between the two treatment groups, casting significant doubt on the efficacy of vertebral augmentation procedures. The American Academy of Orthopaedic

Surgeons subsequently published guidelines with a strong recommendation against the use of vertebroplasty and a weak recommendation for kyphoplasty.[5] This led to withdrawal of coverage for these procedures by insurance payors and a precipitous drop in the number performed in subsequent years.[6]

However, several criticisms have been made regarding the design of the *NEJM* studies,[7–13] including: (1) enrollment difficulties leading them to liberalize the inclusion criteria to patients with Visual Analogue Scale (VAS) pain scores as low as 3/10; (2) selection bias due to a significant proportion of eligible patients not wishing to be randomized and thus declining to participate; (3) inclusion criteria which did not include physical exam findings, leading to concerns that patients may have had back pain that did not correlate with the area of the fracture; (4) concern that patients with chronic fractures were included in the study; (5) the sham-procedure control arm included an injection of local anesthetic to the periosteum or facet and thus might have had a therapeutic effect; (6) high crossover from control to treatment group; and (7) a lower than clinically effective amount of cement was injected. The publication of these trials has led to incredible controversy over the use of vertebroplasty and kyphoplasty, which additional randomized-controlled trials (RCTs) have attempted to address.

Farrokhi et al. performed a single-blinded trial of 82 patients randomized to either vertebroplasty or optimal medical management.[14] The study included those with point-tenderness at the level of fracture; those with painless fractures were excluded. They reported improved pain and quality of life scores with vertebro-plasty, which were maintained up to 24 months postop. At 36 months, quality of life scores favored vertebroplasty, while pain scores were not significantly different between the groups. In another RCT with 125 patients, Blasco et al. concluded that patients treated with vertebroplasty had significantly improved pain scores at 2 months compared to conservative management, but that vertebroplasty and conservative management were equally effective at 1 year.[15] In a meta-analysis published in 2013 by Anderson et al., vertebral augmentation resulted in improved pain relief, functional recovery, and quality of life scores compared to conservative or sham treatment at 6 and 12 months follow-up.[16]

Though the majority of vertebral compression fractures will heal and resolve on their own, it is likely that there is a subpopulation where vertebral augmen-tation is advantageous over conservative treatment, by providing faster relief of pain and return to function. These may involve patients with pain that does not improve after a period of conservative treatment (perhaps 6 weeks, but this has yet to be clearly defined in the literature), mechanical pain, focal tenderness corresponding to the location of the fracture, and a fracture pattern that is less likely to heal. Further studies are required to define with greater certainty the characteristics of this subgroup that would benefit the most from vertebral augmentation procedures.

REFERENCES

1. Wardlaw D, Cummings SR, Van Meirhaeghe J, et al. Efficacy and safety of balloon kyphoplasty compared with non-surgical care for vertebral compression fracture (FREE): A randomised controlled trial. *Lancet.* 2009; 373: 1016–1024.
2. Klazen CAH, Lohle PNM, De Vries J, et al. Vertebroplasty versus conservative treatment in acute osteoporotic vertebral compression fractures (vertos II): An open-label randomized trial. *Lancet.* 2010; 376: 1085–1092.
3. Buchbinder R, Osborne RH, Ebeling PR, et al. A randomized trial of vertebroplasty for painful osteoporotic vertebral fractures. *NEJM.* 2009; 361(6): 557–568.
4. Kallmes DF, Comstock BA, Heagerty PJ, et al. A randomized trial of vertebroplasty for osteoporotic spinal fractures. *NEJM.* 2009; 361(6): 569–579.
5. Esses SI, McGuire R, Jenkins J, et al. American Academy of Orthopaedic Surgeons clinical practice guideline on the treatment of osteoporotic spinal compression fractures. *JBJS Am.* 2011; 93(20): 1934–1936.
6. Sayari AJ, Liu Y, Raphael Cohen J, et al. Trends in vertebroplasty and kyphoplasty after thoracolumbar osteoporotic fracture: A large database study from 2005 to 2012. *J Orthop.* 2015; 12: S217–S222.
7. Bono C, Heggeness M, Mick C, Resnick D, Watters WC. North American Spine Society: Newly released vertebroplasty randomized controlled trials: A tale of two trials. *Spine J.* 2010; 10: 238–240.
8. Buchbinder R, Kallmes D. Vertebroplasty: When randomized placebo-controlled trial results clash with common belief. *Spine J.* 2010; 10: 241–243.
9. Vlahos A, Sewall LE. An objection to the *New England Journal of Medicine* vertebroplasty articles. *Can Assoc Radiol J.* 2010; 61: 121–122.
10. Boszczyk B. Volume matters: A review of procedural details of two randomized controlled vertebroplasty trials of 2009. *Eur Spine J.* 2010; 19: 1837–1840.
11. Munk PL. Vertebroplasy: Where do we go from here? *Skeletal Radiol.* 2011; 40: 371–373.
12. O'Toole JE, Traynelis VC. Vertebral compression fractures. *J Neurosurg Spine.* 2011; 14: 555–560.
13. Chen L, Black C, Hirsch JA, Beall D, Munk P, Murphy K, et al. Vertebroplasty trials: The medium is the message. *JVIR.* 2014; 25(2): 323–325.
14. Farrokhi MR, Alibai E, Maghami Z. Randomized controlled trial of percutaneous vertebroplasty versus optimal medical management for the relief of pain and disability in acute osteoporotic vertebral compression fractures. *J Neurosurg Spine* 2011; 14: 561–569.
15. Blasco, et al. Effect of vertebroplasty on pain relief, quality of life, and the incidence of new vertebral fractures: A 12-month randomized follow-up, controlled trial. *J Bone Miner Res.* 2012; 27(5): 1159–1166.
16. Anderson PA, Froyshteter AB, Tontz WL Jr. Meta-analysis of vertebral augmentation compared with conservative treatment for osteoporotic spinal fractures. *J Bone Miner Res.* 2013; 28(2): 372–382.

The Subaxial Cervical Spine Injury Classification System: A Novel Approach to Recognize the Importance of Morphology, Neurology, and Integrity of the Disco-Ligamentous Complex*

Vaccaro AR, Hurlbert R. John, et al. Spine 32:2365–2374, 2007

Reviewed by Jonathan W. Riffle and Christopher M. Maulucci

Research Question/Objective   Injuries to the spinal column are frequently seen by trauma surgeons, with trauma to the subaxial cervical spine accounting for almost 50% of all spine injuries and the vast majority of spinal cord injuries. Classification systems prior to this study were based on an assumed mechanism of injury implied from plain radiographs and did not take into account ligamentous structure integrity and neurologic status. No "gold standard" of classifying cervical spine injury existed, and systems varied even between surgeons at the same institution. The primary goal of this study was to identify a novel classification system for subaxial cervical spine injuries based on three components. The classification system was designed to provide a uniform system of classifying injuries and an algorithm in which to guide treatment.

Study Design   The classification system was derived through a literature review and expert opinion of experienced spine surgeons from a subcommittee of the Spine Trauma Study Group (STSG). In addition, a multicenter reliability and validity study of the system was conducted on a collection of trauma cases presented to spine surgeons.

Sample Size   Twenty spine surgeons given 11 cervical trauma cases.

Follow-Up   Not applicable.

---

* Vaccaro AR, Hurlbert RJ, et al. A Novel Approach to Recognize the Importance of Morphology, Neurology, and Integrity of the Disco-Ligamentous Complex. *Spine.* 2007; 32: 2365–2374.

Inclusion/Exclusion Criteria   This criterion was not described in the study.

Intervention   Not applicable.

Results   Three primary injury characteristics were identified: injury morphology as determined by the pattern of spinal column disruption on imaging studies, integrity of the disco-ligamentous complex, and neurologic status of the patient. These three injury characteristics were recognized as independent predictors of clinical outcome. Each category contains subgroups, which are assigned a point total and graded from least to most severe. The overall numerical value assists in the decision to pursue nonoperative versus operative treatment of the cervical injury. The greater the point total in the subgroup, the more severe the injury.

Injury morphology is characterized as no overt abnormality (0 points), simple compression (1 point), burst (2 points), distraction (3 points), and rotation/translation (4 points). Compressive injuries are defined as loss of height through a portion or all of a vertebral body. Nondisplaced or minimally displaced lateral mass or facet fractures are categorized under compressive injuries unless there is visible translation seen on imaging. Distractive injuries are categorized by evidence of anatomic dissociation in the vertical axis. Distraction injuries involve ligamentous disruption through the disc space or facet joints. Examples include facet subluxation or dislocation. Other injury patterns that fall under this category include hyperextension injuries where there is disruption of the anterior longitudinal ligament and widening of the intervertebral disc space. Due to the magnitude of force required to generate a distractive injury, these injuries tend to confer a great deal of potential instability of the cervical spine. The imaging modality of choice to identify these occasionally subtle injuries is magnetic resonance imagining (MRI). Translation/rotation injuries are graded the most severe of all the injury morphologies and are defined as radiographic evidence of horizontal displacement of one portion of the subaxial cervical spine with respect to the other. This mechanism may be seen on either static or dynamic imaging sequences. Greater than or equal to 11 degrees of rotation is considered unstable, while 3.5 mm or more of translation is defined as unstable. Examples of translation injuries include unilateral or bilateral facet fracture dislocations, fracture separation of the lateral masses, and bilateral pedicle fractures. This injury morphology almost certainly implies disruption to both the anterior and posterior structures.

The scoring scale for the disco-ligamentous complex (DLC) is as follows: intact (0 points), indeterminate (1 point), and disruption (2 points). The intervertebral disc, anterior and posterior longitudinal ligaments, ligamentum flavum, interspinous and supraspinous ligaments, and facet capsules all fall under this category. The DLC provides restraint against deforming forces while simultaneously allowing fluid movement under normal physiologic loads. The stability of the spine is directly proportional to the integrity of these soft tissues. Furthermore, bone healing after trauma or injury is more predictable than soft tissue healing. If these soft tissues are damaged, progressive instability and deformity could ensue, potentially leading to significant impairment and paralysis. Due to the aforementioned factors, thorough scrutiny of the DLC is paramount in surgical decision making. The DLC is assessed most commonly indirectly via imaging. Imaging may show a widened interspinous space, dislocation or separation of facet joints, subluxation of vertebral bodies, or widening of the disc space. Therefore, distraction and translation injuries are almost always associated with DLC compromise. The strongest portion of the posterior tension band are the facet joint capsules, while the strongest anterior ligamentous structure is the anterior longitudinal ligament. Abnormal facet alignment characterized as articular apposition less than 50% or separation over 2 mm through the facet joint is an absolute sign of DLC injury. Another absolute indicator of DLC disruption is abnormal widening of the anterior disc space seen on neutral or extension radiographs. MRI studies may show hyperintensity on T2 sequences through the disc space, indicating increased fluid content. This increased fluid content is indicative of edema that correlates to disc or annulus disruption. Finally, the interspinous ligament is the weakest of all ligaments in the subaxial cervical spine. Imaging may show interspinous widening or splaying of the spinous processes, but DLC compromise is only assumed if lateral flexion radiographs demonstrate abnormal facet alignment or an angulation of greater than or equal to 11 degrees at the said vertebral interspace.

Neurologic status is graded as intact (0 points), root injury (1 point), complete cord injury (2 points), incomplete cord injury (3 points). An additional 1 point is added for continuous cord compression with a neurologic deficit. Up until this scoring system, neurologic status was not a component of any of the widely used trauma classification systems. The nerves and spinal cord are generally well protected in the spinal column, and a neurological injury infers that the subaxial spine has received a significant force leading to potential instability. Furthermore, neurologic status may be considered the most influential predictor of treatment. Incomplete injuries in a patient with root or cord compression usually warrant a decompressive procedure to allow the patient the greatest chance of neural recovery.

To fully classify an injury utilizing the Subaxial Cervical Spine Injury Classification (SLIC) scale, the injury axes (morphology, DLC, and neurologic status) as well as the spinal level involved, a bony injury description, and confounders are added. These provide a descriptive interpretation of the injury that all clinicians may apply to the assessment and treatment of subaxial cervical spine injuries. Bony injury descriptors include fractures or dislocations of specific portions of the bony elements of the subaxial spine. Confounders include systemic diseases that confer inherent or potential spinal instability. In trauma cases involving multiple levels, a SLIC score is calculated for each level.

Patients with scores of 1–3 can be treated nonoperatively, patients with 4 points can be treated nonsurgically or surgically, according to surgeons' preference and patients' condition, and patients with five or more points are referred to surgery, with the realignment, neurological decompression (if indicated), and stabilization.[1]

Twenty members of the 30 selected surgeons completed the second analysis of the 11 trauma cases after 6 weeks. The 11 cases were analyzed with the SLIC system as well as the Ferguson and Allen et al.[2] and Harris[3] systems during both stages of analysis. The current study shows moderate reliability of the SLIC scale, which will improve when the scale is better understood. Construct validity also showed a high degree of agreement. Construct validity was assessed by comparing the numerical SLIC score to participants' assessment of whether the case was surgical or nonsurgical. Raters agreed with the SLIC algorithm in 91.8% of cases. Construct validity is also expected improve with further testing.

Study Limitations   While this study utilizes an algorithm determining which injuries are operative versus nonoperative, the study does not delve into the specific operative techniques used to treat the injuries. Nor does the SLIC system recommend an operative approach, that is, anterior, posterior, or combined. The study also demonstrated a limited sample size and only examined 11 cases. More cases would have to be analyzed in order to further increase the power and the validity of the study. Furthermore, only 30 surgeons judged the study. A greater number of clinicians and surgeons would need to be involved in order to further validate the study. Within the three axes examined, morphology, DLC, and neurologic status, DLC showed the lowest interrater and intrarater intraclass correlation (ICC) results. Interrater ICC was 0.49, and intrarater was 0.66. This is in part due to the difficulty in objectifying DLC compromise. For example, an imaging study could show normal spinal alignment, but an MRI study could show hyperintensity in the disc space, facet capsule, or interspinous ligament. It is clear that a pathological process exists based upon MRI imaging, but the clinical significance is not clear. The SLIC scale attempts to address this problem by assigning the DLC status as *indeterminate* until the clinical significance is fully elucidated (see Table 18.1). Further research will need to be undertaken in order to better define DLC status. There was also only moderate reliability in the interrater ICC of the morphology axis, with ICC of 0.57. The disagreement between reviewers is most likely in the conversion of nonuniform, descriptive systems to the SLIC system. Prior classification systems often contained large numbers of morphologic descriptors, whereas the current SLIC system contains only a few. For example, the Ferguson and Allen system describes compressive flexion and vertical compression as two separate entities. In the SLIC system, they are both considered compression morphology. It is thought that, with greater exposure to the SLIC system, there will be greater interrater reliability for this axis.

Table 18.1   SLIC: Subaxial Injury Classification

Characteristics	Points
Injury morphology	
No abnormality	0
Compression	1
Burst	2
Distraction	3
Translation	4
Integrity of the disco-ligamentous complex	
Intact	0
Indeterminate	1
Disrupted	2
Neurological status	
Intact	0
Nerve root injury	1
Complete	2
Incomplete	3
Persistent cord compression	+1

Relevant Studies   The prior classification systems, which have been widely used, are the Ferguson and Allen system and the Harris system. The Ferguson and Allen system consisted of six categories that are based upon the radiographic appearance of the subaxial cervical spine. The mechanism of injury was inferred from the recoil position seen on the radiographs. The Harris system included rotational vectors in flexion and extension, and excluded the distractive forces seen in the Ferguson and Allen system. Both systems only categorized a variety of anatomic fracture patterns into arbitrary compartments. Neither system takes into account the potential for ligamentous injury or neurologic deficit. Furthermore, both demonstrated low reliability scores. The Allen classification of subaxial spinal injury is not recommended for describing the mechanistic and imaging findings in cervical spine and spinal cord injury due to its low reliability, ICC of 0.53.[4] Finally, the Harris classification of subaxial spinal injury is not recommended for describing the bony and soft tissue characteristics seen on imaging studies in spinal cord injury due to its low reliability, ICC of 0.42.[4] As stated earlier, the SLIC scale guides the physician to either operative or nonoperative treatment, but it lacks the choice of surgical approach. A study by Dvorak et al.[5] utilizes the SLIC scale and provides an evidence-based algorithm for specific surgical approaches concerning injuries to the subaxial cervical spine, which may assist surgeons in their decision-making process.

REFERENCES

1. Joaquim AF, Patel AA, Vacaro A. Cervical injuries scored according to the Subaxial Injury Classification system: An analysis of the literature. *J Craniovertebr Junction Spine*. 2014; 5: 65–70.
2. Allen BL, Ferguson RL, Lehmann TR, O'Brien RP. A mechanistic classification of closed, indirect fractures and dislocations of the lower cervical spine. *Spine*. 1982; 7: 1–27.
3. Harris JH Jr., Edeiken-Monroe B, Kopaniky DR. A practical classification of acute cervical spine injuries. *Orthop Clin North Am*. 1986; 17: 15–30.
4. Aarabi B, Walters B, Dhall SS, et al. Subaxial cervial spine injury classification systems. *Neurosurgery*. 2013; 72: 170–186.
5. Dvorak M, Fisher C, Fehlings MG, et al. The surgical approach to subaxial cervical spine injuries: An evidence-based algorithm based on the SLIC classification system. *Spine*. 2007; 32: 2620–2629.

Early versus Delayed Decompression for Traumatic Cervical Spinal Cord Injury: Results of the Surgical Timing in Acute Spinal Cord Injury Study (STASCIS)*

Fehlings MG, Vaccaro A, Wilson JR, et al. PLoS One 7(2):e32037, 2012

Reviewed by Jeffrey A. Rihn, Joseph T. Labrum IV, and Theresa Clark Rihn

Research Question/Objective Although significant preclinical evidence exists that supports early surgical intervention in acute spinal cord injury, the effect of timely surgical decompression on clinical outcome remains a matter of debate. The central aim of this study was to evaluate the effect of early surgical decompression, defined as occurring less than 24 hours after injury, versus late surgical decompression, defined as occurring over 24 hours after injury, on postoperative neurologic outcomes following traumatic cervical spinal cord injuries.

Study Design This study was a prospective cohort study performed across six North American centers specializing in spinal cord trauma that evaluated adult patients with acute cervical spinal cord injuries (SCIs) that were surgically decompressed before or after the 24-hour post-SCI time point. The primary outcome for this study was ordinal change observed in ASIA Impairment Scale (AIS) grade at 6 months postoperative follow-up. Baseline AIS grades were obtained within 24 hours of SCI in all study patients. Secondary outcome measures included complication rates and mortality of both treatment groups.

Sample Size This study screened 470 potentialparticipants and enrolled 313 patients into the study who met inclusion and exclusion criteria. Of this sample, 182 patients underwent early decompression and 131 underwent late surgical decompression.

---

* Fehlings MG, Vaccaro A, Wilson JR, et al. Early versus delayed decompression for traumatic cervical spinal cord injury: Results of the Surgical Timing in Acute Spinal Cord Injury Study (STASCIS). *PLoS One.* 2012; 7(2): e32037.

Follow-Up Study follow-up occurred at 6 months postoperatively, at which time AIS grades were again recorded. Secondary outcome measures included complication rates and mortality.

Inclusion/Exclusion Criteria Criteria for patient inclusion in this cohort study were outlined as adults aged 16–80 with acute cervical spinal cord compression injury between vertebral levels C2 and T1 confirmed by magnetic resonance imaging (MRI) or computed tomography (CT) myelography with initial Glascow Coma Scale score >13 and initial AIS grades A–D. Additionally, the patient or proxy had to provide consent for enrollment into the study. Exclusion criteria for the study included (1) cognitive impairment preventing accurate neurologic assessment, (2) penetrating injuries to the neck, (3) pregnant females, (4) preinjury neurologic deficits or disease, (5) life-threatening injuries that prevent early decompression of the spinal cord, (6) arrival at health center >24 hours after SCI, and (7) surgery >7 days after SCI.

Intervention Early surgical decompression, defined as occurring less than 24 hours after cervical spinal cord injury, versus late surgical decompression, defined as occurring over 24 hours after traumatic cervical spinal cord injury.

Results

Sampling: This study screened 470 potential participants and enrolled 313 patients, of which 182 underwent early surgical decompression and 131 underwent late surgical decompression. During the 6-month prospective period, 5 patients died (4 early intervention, 1 late intervention), and 86 patients were lost to follow-up (47 early intervention, 39 late intervention). In total, 222 patients, composed of 131 patients in the early intervention cohort and 91 patients in the late intervention cohort, completed 6-month postoperative follow-up evaluation for postintervention AIS grading.

Cohort Demographics: Cohort demographic analysis showed a significant difference in age and baseline AIS grades across cohorts. The early surgery group was significantly younger, with a mean age of 45.0 ± 17.2 years, while the late intervention cohort had a mean age of 50.7 ± 15.9 years ($p < 0.01$). Neurologic status on admission, assessed with baseline AIS grades, showed significant difference between study groups, with AIS grades A and B being more common in the early intervention cohort, and AIS grades C and D were more common in the late intervention cohort ($p < 0.01$). All other demographic variables analyzed, including gender, etiology of SCI, Charlson co-morbidity index, and Glasgow Coma Scale showed no significant difference across study groups.

Cohort Interventions: Mean time to surgical decompression for the early and late intervention cohorts was 14.2 ($\pm$ 5.4) hours and 48.3 ($\pm$ 29.3) hours, respectively, with this difference being statistically significant ($p < 0.01$). A significantly higher proportion of the patients enrolled in the early intervention cohort received steroids at hospital admission when compared to the late intervention cohort ($p = 0.04$).

Neurologic Recovery: A significant improvement in AIS grades was seen at 6-month follow-up across the entire study population ($p = 0.02$). At 6-month follow-up, 74 patients in the early intervention group (56.5%) and 45 patients in the late intervention group (49.5%) experienced at least a 1-grade improvement in AIS scoring. After controlling for preoperative neurologic status and steroid administration, calculation of an odds ratio for a 1-grade improvement for early versus late intervention was calculated as 1.38 (95% CI: 0.74–2.57). A 2-grade ordinal improvement in AIS at 6-month follow-up was seen in 26 patients in the early intervention group (19.8%) and in 8 patients in the late intervention group (8.8%), with an early versus late intervention odds ratio of 2.83 (95% CI: 1.10–7.28).

Complications and Mortality: Across the 313 patients enrolled in the study, 97 major postoperative complications occurred in 84 of patients, experienced by 44 patients in the early intervention cohort and 40 patients in the late intervention cohort. There was no significant difference found in postoperative complications between the early and late intervention cohorts ($p = 0.21$). During the 6-month prospective period, four patients in the early intervention cohort and one late patient in the late intervention cohort died.

Study Limitations   Overall, 27% of enrolled study participants were lost to 6-month follow-up and therefore a significant proportion of 6-month postintervention AIS grades could not be assessed. The early and late intervention cohorts did display some significant differences in baseline characteristics, which may have introduced bias into the study results. The early surgical decompression cohort had a significantly greater proportion of patients presenting with more severely impaired neurologic status as assessed with baseline AIS grades upon admission when compared to the late intervention cohort. The early surgical decompression cohort also had a significantly lower mean age when compared to the late surgical decompression cohort. Furthermore, analysis of interventions administered across groups showed a significantly higher rate of steroid administration at hospital admission to the early intervention group when compared to the late intervention group ($p = 0.04$).

The authors of this study postulated that the significantly worse neurologic status, significantly younger age, and significantly increased proportion of steroid administration seen in the early intervention cohort when compared to the late intervention cohort was likely a result of (1) participating surgeons treating younger patients with severe presentations of SCI more aggressively, and/or (2) younger patients presented with less comorbidities, allowing for accelerated medical stabilization and subsequent surgical intervention. Either may have resulted in an inherent selection bias with cohort assignments.

A large randomized controlled trial analyzing the effect of early versus late surgical decompression in traumatic SCI would be superior to a prospective cohort analysis, but it is not feasible in this patient population due to practical and ethical dilemmas.

Relevant Studies   Prior to this study, laboratory studies found significant evidence supporting a secondary injury mechanism that was propagated over time of spinal cord compression and advocated that early surgical intervention would preempt these pathologic changes and result in better neurologic outcomes.[1–8] Clinical studies did not initially find significant evidence to support this theory, but time intervals adopted for the definition of early versus late surgical intervention were 72 hours.[9,10] A systematic review on early versus late surgical decompression reported that surgical decompression prior to 24 hours post-SCI resulted in improved outcomes compared to later decompression and conservative treatment.[11] With uncertainty in optimal timing to surgical intervention following SCI, the Spine Trauma Study Group carried out a literature review and designated 8–24 hours post-SCI as the interval for early surgical decompression.[12] The authors of this study adopted this metric for early intervention into their study construct, and evidence suggests this time line is better aligned for the prevention of secondary injury mechanisms following SCI and improved neurologic outcomes.

In a subgroup analysis of the STASCIS data, Wilson et al. published a clinical prediction model for complications following traumatic spinal cord injury.[13] A greater likelihood of complications during the hospitalization following acute traumatic spinal cord injury was associated with the following indicators: (1) lack of steroid administration on admission, (2) severe AIS grade at presentation, (3) high-energy injury mechanisms, (4) older age, and (5) higher frequency of significant comorbidity.[13]

Recently, Furlan et al. performed a cost-utility analysis utilizing the data collected from STASCIS.[14] This analysis determined that early spinal decompression is more cost-effective compared to the delayed spinal decompression for patients with both incomplete and complete motor deficit.[14]

As a randomized controlled trial likely cannot be carried out to address this clinical question, this study provides the best evidence to date analyzing the effect of early versus late surgical decompression following traumatic cervical spine injuries, validating prior hypotheses that early intervention is associated with significantly improved neurologic outcomes.

REFERENCES

1. Brodkey J, Richards D, Blasingame J, et al. Reversible spinal cord trauma in cats: Additive effects of direct pressure and ischemia. *J Neurosurgery*. 1972; 37(5): 591–593.
2. Carlson GD, Minato Y, Okada A, et al. Early time-dependent decompression for spinal cord injury: Vascular mechanisms of recovery. *J Neurotrauma*. 1997; 14(12): 951–962.
3. Delamarter RB, Sherman J, Carr JB. Pathophysiology of spinal cord injury: Recovery after immediate and delayed decompression. *J Bone Joint Surg Am*. 1995; 77(7): 1042–1049.
4. Dimar JR, Glassman SD, Raque GH, et al. The influence of spinal canal narrowing and timing of decompression on neurologic recovery after spinal cord contusion in a rat model. *Spine*. 1999; 24(16): 1623–1633.
5. Dolan EJ, Tator CH, Endrenyi L. The value of decompression for acute experimental spinal cord compression injury. *J Neurosurg*. 1980; 53(6): 749–755.
6. Guha A, Tator CH, Endrenyi L, et al. Decompression of the spinal cord improves recovery after acute experimental spinal cord compression injury. *Paraplegia*. 1987; 25(4): 324–339.
7. Tarlov IM. Spinal cord compression studies. III. Time limits for recovery after gradual compression in dogs. *AMA Arch Neurol Psychiatry*. 1954; 71(5): 588–597.
8. Carlson GD, Gorden CD, Oliff HS, et al. Sustained spinal cord compression: Part I: Time-dependent effect on long-term pathophysiology. *J Bone Joint Surg Am*. 2003; 85(1): 86–94.
9. McKinley W, Meade MA, Kirshblum S, et al. Outcomes of early surgical management versus late or no surgical intervention after acute spinal cord injury. *Arch Phys Med Rehabil*. 2004; 85(11): 1818–1825.
10. Vaccaro AR, Daugherty RJ, Sheehan TP, et al. Neurologic outcome of early versus late surgery for cervical spinal cord injury. *Spine*. 1997; 22(22): 609–612.
11. LaRosa G, Conti A, Cardali S, et al. Does early decompression improve neurological outcome of spinal cord injured patients? Appraisal of the literature using a meta-analytical approach. *Spinal Cord*. 2004; 42(9): 503–512.
12. Fehlings MG, Rabin D, Sears W, et al. Current practice in the timing of surgical intervention in spinal cord injury. *Spine*. 2010; 35(21): 166–173.
13. Wilson JR, Arnold PM, Singh A, Kalsi-Ryan S, Fehlings MG. Clinical prediction model for acute inpatient complications after traumatic cervical spinal cord injury: A subanalysis from the Surgical Timing in Acute Spinal Cord Injury Study. *J Neurosurg Spine*. 2012; 17(1 Suppl): 46–51, doi: 10.3171/2012.4.AOSPINE 1246.
14. Furlan JC, Craven BC, Massicotte EM, Fehlings MG. Early versus delayed surgical decompression of spinal cord after traumatic cervical spinal cord injury: A cost-utility analysis. *World Neurosurgery*, 2016; 88: 166–174.

CHAPTER 20

The Canadian C-Spine Rule versus the NEXUS Low-Risk Criteria in Patients with Trauma*

Stiell IG, Clement CM, McKnight RD, et al. N Engl J Med 349:2510–2518, 2003

Reviewed by Theodore J. Steelman and Melvin D. Helgeson

Research Question/Objective   Due to the tremendous volume of trauma patients seen every year in emergency departments who are at risk for cervical spine injury, a reliable decision rule to guide the responsible use of radiology resources with an emphasis on avoiding missed injuries is required. The goal of this study was to evaluate and compare two commonly used guidelines: the Canadian C-Spine (cervical-spine) Rule (CCR) and the National Emergency X-Radiography Utilization Study (NEXUS) Low-Risk Criteria (NLC) decision rules.

Study Design   This prospective cohort study was conducted in the emergency departments of nine Canadian tertiary medical centers with a total of 394 participating physicians. Eligible patients were evaluated using both the CCR and NLC decision rules. For a patient to be considered "low risk" and not warrant imaging per the NLC, he or she must meet all five of the following criteria: no tenderness at the posterior midline of the cervical spine; no focal neurologic deficit; a normal level of alertness; no evidence of intoxication; and no clinically apparent, painful injury that might distract the patient from the pain of a cervical-spine injury. CCR criteria are listed separately in Figure 20.1. Seventy percent of eligible patients underwent cervical spine imaging (70% determined by hospital policy). The remaining patients were evaluated by the Proxy Outcome Assessment Tool, a phone questionnaire previously determined to be 100% sensitive for identifying cervical spine injury.[1] The primary outcome was any clinically important cervical spine injury defined as any fracture, dislocation, or ligamentous instability demonstrated by imaging. Isolated, nonclinically important fractures were osteophyte avulsion,

---

* Stiell IG, Clement CM, McKnight RD, et al. The Canadian C-spine rule versus the NEXUS low-risk criteria in patients with trauma. *N Engl J Med*. 2003; 349: 2510–2518.

transverse process not involving a facet joint, a spinous process not involving lamina, or simple vertebral compression of less than 25% of body height.

Sample Size   Enrollments numbered 8283 patients, of which 7438 patients had complete information as directed by the CCR and NLC decision rules. In 845 of the 8283 patients, physicians did not evaluate range of motion as indicated by the CCR and were assessed as "intermediate."

Follow-Up   Thirty percent of the study population did not have X-rays taken and were assessed via phone call 14 days after their respective emergency room visit using the Proxy Outcome Assessment Tool.

Inclusion/Exclusion Criteria   For patients to be considered for enrollment, they had to have been age 16 or over with trauma within the previous 48 hours to the head or neck. Eligible patients were both in stable condition and met all of the following criteria: (1) visible injury above the clavicles, (2) nonambulatory, and (3) a dangerous mechanism of injury. Dangerous mechanism was defined as a fall from an elevation ≥ 3 feet or 5 stairs, an axial load to the head (e.g., diving), a motor vehicle collision at high speed (>100 km/hr) or with rollover or ejection, a collision involving a motorized recreational vehicle, or a bicycle collision. Patients were not considered eligible if they were under the age of 16 years; had penetrating neck trauma, acute paralysis, or known vertebral disease; had been evaluated previously for the same injury; or were pregnant.

Intervention   Not applicable.

Results   Of the 8283 enrolled patients, 169 (2.0%) demonstrated clinically important cervical-spine injuries. Physicians did not evaluate range of motion in 845 (10.2%) of the patients contrary to the CCR; these cases were classified as "indeterminate." Analyses that excluded these "indeterminate" cases found that the CCR was more sensitive than the NLC (99.4% versus 90.7%, $p < 0.001$) and more specific (45.1% versus 36.8%, $p < 0.001$) for injury and would have resulted in lower cervical spine imaging rates (55.9% versus 66.6%, $p < 0.001$). In secondary analyses that included all patients, the sensitivity and specificity of CCR, assuming that the indeterminate cases were all positive, were 99.4% and 40.4%, respectively ($p < 0.001$ for both comparisons with the NLC). Assuming that the CCR was negative for all indeterminate cases, these rates were 95.3% ($p = 0.09$ for the comparison with the NLC) and 50.7% ($p = 0.001$). The CCR would have missed one patient and the NLC would have missed 16 patients with important injuries.

Study Limitations   All 394 physicians involved in patient enrollment and assessment received a 1-hour training session. There was a lack of posttraining knowledge assessment and relative complexity of the CCR compared to the NLC; the CCR is based on three high-risk criteria, five low-risk criteria, and the ability of patients to rotate their necks compared to the NLC, which has five criteria without range of motion (ROM) testing. This increase in algorithm complexity is evidenced by the 10% nonadherence to the CCR algorithm of ROM testing despite lower than average actual injury within that patient subset (0.8% versus 2% overall seen in the study). Some authors are critical of the NLC exclusion criteria such as "no distracting painful injuries," "no evidence of intoxication," and "no focal neurological deficit" because these items have the potential for variability in their interpretation and decreased interobserver reliability, despite efforts by the NEXUS working group and others to define these criteria clearly.[2-6] In this study, only 70% of the patients went on to receive imaging to verify or refute the clinical guideline decision making; however, the remaining 30% were determined not to have a clinically significant injury by way of a Proxy Outcome Assessment Tool, which was developed and validated at only one point by same group that developed it and has not been validated elsewhere.[1]

Summary of Limitations
- Physician training on algorithm use.
- Exclusion criteria somewhat vague.
- Final determination of the injury may not be clinically relevant.

Relevant Studies   Initial development of the NLC was based on a retrospective review of prospectively collected data by Hoffman et al. at the UCLA Emergency Medicine Center looking at 974 patients with 27 cervical spine fractures. Results of their 5-point criteria, they stated, would have led to identification of all 27 fractures and a reduction in film ordering by 37%.[7] This initial study was validated by the NEXUS group in a prospective observation multicenter study involving 21 centers and 34,069 patients across the United States. The NLC decision rules instrument identified all but 8 (2 of which were deemed "clinically significant") of the 818 patients who had cervical-spine injury, with 99.0% sensitivity and a negative predictive value of 99.8%. In that series, radiographic imaging would have been avoided in 4309 patients (12.6%).[3] Interobserver agreement for the decision instrument as a whole was found to have substantial agreement, with a kappa of 0.73.[6]

The Canadian C-Spine Rule was derived from a prospective cohort study at 10 large Canadian community and university hospitals evaluating 20 standardized clinical findings prior to radiography.[8] The patient sample consisted of 8924 adults demonstrating 151 (1.7%) important cervical-spine injuries. Again, nearly 70% (68.9%) of the study cohort had X-rays taken to confirm or refute clinical exam findings, with the remaining cohort evaluated with the Proxy Outcome Assessment Tool. They found the CCR to have 100% sensitivity and 42.5% specificity for identifying 151 clinically important cervical-spine injuries, with a potential cervical-spine ordering rate of 58.2% from 68.9%, a reduction of 15.5%. Subsequent validation in the UK emergency department setting found the CCR to have an substantial interobserver reliability, with a kappa of 0.75.[9]

In 2007, Duane et al. presented their results looking to validate the NLC using CT as the *gold standard*. Over a 1-year period, they prospectively assessed 534 blunt trauma patients at a Level 1 trauma center and found 52 patients with fracture, of which 40 were identified using the NLC guidelines, for a sensitivity of 76.9% and a negative predictive value of 95.7%.[10] Similarly, the same group published their results in 2011, validating the CCR using CT as the *gold standard*, with 3201 blunt trauma patients over the age of 16. They ultimately found 192 patients with cervical-spine fractures, of which the CCR demonstrated a sensitivity of CCS was 100% as was negative predictive value.[11] While these results are considerably different than seen previously, especially in the case of the NEXUS criteria, the cause may be a combination of smaller sample size compared to prior validation studies as well as increased sensitivity of the *gold standard*, in this case CT, to evaluate for previously missed fractures (Figure 20.1).

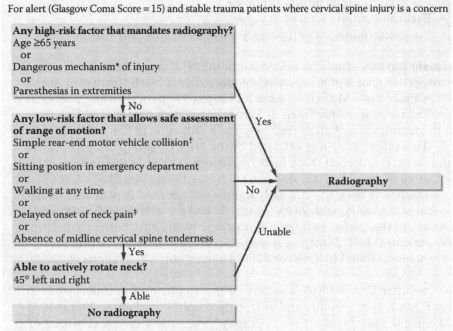

For alert (Glasgow Coma Score = 15) and stable trauma patients where cervical spine injury is a concern

Any high-risk factor that mandates radiography?
Age ≥65 years
or
Dangerous mechanism* of injury
or
Paresthesias in extremities
↓ No

Any low-risk factor that allows safe assessment of range of motion?
Simple rear-end motor vehicle collision†
or
Sitting position in emergency department
or
Walking at any time
or
Delayed onset of neck pain†
or
Absence of midline cervical spine tenderness
↓ Yes

Able to actively rotate neck?
45° left and right
↓ Able

No radiography

Yes

No → **Radiography**

Unable

Rule not applicable if: Nontrauma cases, Glasgow Coma Score <15, unstable vital signs, age <16 years, acute paralysis, known vertebral disease, or previous surgery of cervical spine.

*Fall from elevation ≥0.9, (3 feet)/5 stairs, axial load to head—for example, diving, motor vehicle collision high speed (>100 km/h), rollover, ejection, motorized recreational vehicles, bicycle struck, or collision.

†Excludes: Pushed into oncoming traffic, hit by bus or large truck, rollover, hit by high-speed vehicle.

‡Not immediate onset of neck pain.

Figure 20.1 Canadian C-spine rule. (Reprinted from Stiell IG, et al., *BMJ*, 339, b4146, 2009. With permission.)

REFERENCES

1. Vandemheen KL. Validity evaluation of the cervical spine injury Proxy Outcome Assessment Tool in the CCC Study. *Acad Emerg Med.* 1999; 6: 434.
2. Hoffman JR, Mower WR. National Emergency X-radiography Utilization Study: Doing what's right for your patients. *Emerg Med Australasia: EMA.* 2005; 17: 406–407.
3. Hoffman JR, Mower WR, Wolfson AB, Todd KH, Zucker MI. Validity of a set of clinical criteria to rule out injury to the cervical spine in patients with blunt trauma. National Emergency X-Radiography Utilization Study Group. *N Engl J Med.* 2000; 343: 94–99.
4. Hoffman JR, Wolfson AB, Todd K, Mower WR, Grp N. Selective cervical spine radiography in blunt trauma: Methodology of the National Emergency X-Radiography Utilization Study (NEXUS). *Ann Emerg Med.* 1998; 32: 461–469.
5. Heffernan DS, Schermer CR, Lu SW. What defines a distracting injury in cervical spine assessment? *Journal of Trauma-Injury Infection and Critical Care.* 2005; 59: 1396–1399.
6. Mahadevan S, Mower WR, Hoffman JR, Peeples N, Goldberg W, Sonner R. Interrater reliability of cervical spine injury criteria in patients with blunt trauma. *Ann Emerg Med.* 1998; 31: 197–201.
7. Hoffman JR, Schriger DL, Mower W, Luo JS, Zucker M. Low-risk criteria for cervical-spine radiography in blunt trauma: A prospective study. *Ann Emerg Med.* 1992; 21: 1454–1460.
8. Stiell IG, Wells GA, Vandemheen KL, et al. The Canadian C-spine rule for radiography in alert and stable trauma patients. *JAMA.* 2001; 286: 1841–1848.
9. Coffey F, Hewitt S, Stiell I, et al. Validation of the Canadian c-spine rule in the UK emergency department setting. *Emerg Med J.* 2011; 28: 873–876.
10. Duane TM, Dechert T, Wolfe LG, Aboutanos MB, Malhotra AK, Ivatury RR. Clinical examination and its reliability in identifying cervical spine fractures. *J Trauma.* 2007; 62: 1405–1408; discussion 8–10.
11. Duane TM, Wilson SP, Mayglothling J, et al. Canadian cervical spine rule compared with computed tomography: A prospective analysis. *Journal of Trauma-Injury Infection and Critical Care.* 2011; 71: 352–355.

CHAPTER 21

Lumbar Disc Herniation: A Controlled, Prospective Study with 10 Years of Observation

Weber H, et al. Spine 1983

Reviewed by Raj Gala and Peter G. Whang

Research Question/Objective   The type and timing of treatment for lumbar disc herniation remains controversial. The shortcomings of prior studies included concern for information and selection bias, the often retrospective nature of the research, and a lack of diagnostic imaging in the conservatively treated groups. Prior to this study, there was a paucity of randomized controlled trials comparing operative to nonoperative management. Throughout previous nonrandomized comparative studies, the reported outcomes were inconsistent, and there was additional uncertainty surrounding the longevity of treatment effects observed with operative versus nonoperative treatment. The current study aimed to produce more reliable data surrounding the question of operative versus nonoperative treatment for lumbar disc herniation.

Study Design   The main research focus (Group 1) was a prospective, randomized, controlled trial comparing surgery and continued physiotherapy for patients with sciatica secondary to an associated lumbar disc herniation for whom the authors believed there was true equipoise between the two treatments. The study also included two prospective nonrandomized observational arms: a group of patients who were thought to have definitive indications for surgery (Group 2) and a group of patients who were selected for conservative management (Group 3) because they demonstrated continued improvement with initial nonoperative treatment.

Sample Size   The study included 280 consecutive patients with sciatica secondary to a disc herniation. One hundred twenty-six patients were allocated to Group 1 (age range 25 to 55 years) and randomized to either operative treatment (60 patients) or continued physiotherapy (66 patients). Group 2 consisted of 67 patients who were felt to have definitive indications for surgery, and Group 3 included 87 patients who showed continuous improvement during the initial enrollment period and were selected for conservative treatment.

Follow-Up   All patients were sent a questionnaire at 3, 6, and 9 months, as well as 2 and 3 years after enrollment. Patients presented for reexamination at the 1-year and 4-year marks. At 10 years of follow-up, only patients in Group 1 presented for repeat assessment.

Inclusion/Exclusion Criteria   The study included 280 consecutive patients who presented with sciatica with clinical symptoms of L5 or S1 radiculopathy and with corresponding positive findings on radiological investigation (radiculography). Patients were excluded if they had spondylolisthesis or prior operations on the spine. Patients were assigned to definitive surgery (Group 2) if they exhibited any of the following findings: severe and immobile scoliosis, intolerable pain, suddenly occurring and/or progressive muscle weakness, and bladder/rectum paresis. Patients who demonstrated satisfactory progression during the 2-week observational period were allocated into Group 3 to continue nonsurgical treatment. The remaining patients (Group 1) were randomized to either operative or nonoperative management.

Intervention or Treatment Received   All patients were initially admitted to the hospital under the Department of Neurology. Patients who did not require immediate surgery underwent a 14-day observation period of bed rest, medication, and progressive physiotherapy. After this regimen, patients in Group 1 were randomized to either surgery or conservative management. The nonoperative patients were transferred to a rehabilitation hospital for an average of 6 weeks of physiotherapy. Operative patients were placed prone in the knee-elbow position. Ligamentum flavum was excised with resection of the edges of the vertebral arch above and below the exposed interspace, with subsequent nerve root decompression and disc removal. Surgical patients were discharged seven to nine days postoperatively, without further treatment.

Results   Baseline patient characteristics showed a male to female ratio of 1.4:1, similar to prior studies. Twenty-nine percent of the patients were found to have psychosocial problems, a comparable rate to the U.S. general population.

Of the 66 patients who were randomized to conservative treatment, 17 crossed over to operative treatment during the first year (range 1–11 months), with one patient randomized to the surgical group having refused operation. At follow-up, patients were assigned an outcome—good, fair, poor, and bad—according to subjective reports made by the patients. Within the intention-to-treat analysis and as-treated analyses, the 1-year results showed statistically better outcomes in the operated group. By the 4-year mark, the difference was no longer statistically significant, although there remained a trend toward favorable outcomes in the operated group. At final follow-up at 10 years, there was no observable difference between the two groups. "Good" outcomes were reports in 56% of patients initially assigned to conservative treatment compared to 63.6% of patients initially randomized to surgery, but this was not a statistically

Table 21.1 Conservative Treatment Group

	1-Year Results			10-Year Results		
Result	Remained in Original Group	Operated	Total	Remained in Original Group	Operated	Total
Good	16	8	24	27	10	37
Fair	24	4	28	18	7	25
Poor	9	4	13	4	0	4
Bad	0	1	1	0	0	0
Total	49	17	66	49	17	66

Adapted from Weber, H., *Spine*, 1983.

Table 21.2 Operative Treatment Group

	1-Year Results			10-Year Results		
Result	Operated as Planned	Not Operated	Total	Operated as Planned	Not Operated	Total
Good	39	0	39	34	1	35
Fair	15	1	16	16	0	16
Poor	5	0	5	4	0	4
Bad	0	0	0	0	0	0
Total	59	1	60	54	1	55

Adapted from Weber, H., *Spine*, 1983.

significant difference. Tables 21.1 and 21.2 summarize the data for the groups undergoing conservative and operative treatments, respectively.

Muscle weakness was evident in 64 patients prior to randomization. At 10-year follow-up, 5 patients had persistent muscle paresis, which appeared to be unrelated to their treatment group. More than 35% of patients still had sensory deficits at 10 years, equally distributed between the two groups. Otherwise there were no differences in pain and spinal mobility between the two groups at the 10-year follow-up.

Study Limitations   There was a relatively small number of patients who underwent randomization, an issue that is further complicated by the relatively high percentage of crossover (26%) into the operative group. This problem did not appear to significantly affect the statistics because surgical treatment resulted in better outcomes at 1 year on both an intention-to-treat and on an as-treated basis. The research and follow-up were performed by a nonsurgeon, which at least theoretically limited bias toward surgical treatment, but the study was not blinded to patient or researcher. In addition, the researchers used outcome measures that were unique to this study, and they have not been validated in prior or subsequent trials. Another minor weakness relates to the use of radiculography in this study, which is a modality that is now rarely employed to diagnose lumbar disc herniations.

Relevant Studies   A lumbar disc herniation resulting in sciatica is a common cause of discomfort and disability in patients. The natural history of lumbar disc prolapse is typically resolution over time,[1] but there remains debate over the short- and long-term outcomes of surgical treatment. In 2005, Atlas et al.[2] published the long-term results of a prospective cohort series of 400 patients comparing surgical and nonsurgical management of sciatica secondary to lumbar disc herniation. At 10-year follow-up, 69% of patients who underwent discectomy and 61% of patients initially treated nonsurgically ($p = 0.2$) exhibited improvement in their symptoms. There was no difference in work and disability status between the two groups. Nevertheless, there was a statistically higher proportion of surgical patients who reported more complete relief of pain as well as greater satisfaction with their treatment.

The Spine Patient Outcomes Research Trial (SPORT)[3] included 501 patients randomized to either surgical or nonsurgical treatment for symptomatic lumbar disc herniations. While there was significant crossover between groups, according to an intention to treat analysis, patients in both groups demonstrated significant improvements in primary and secondary outcomes over the first 2 years; however, the differences between the two groups were small and not statistically significant. A separate as-treated analysis was also performed because of the high rates of crossover, which showed that the surgical patients did statistically better than nonsurgical patients at all time points during the first 2 years of follow-up. As a continuation of the as-treated analysis, a 4-year follow-up of these same cohorts[4] demonstrated that surgical patients still showed greater improvements in all primary and secondary outcomes except work status compared to those treated nonoperatively. The SPORT study also included a nonrandomized cohort of 743 patients,[5] with 528 electing to proceed with surgery and 191 choosing nonoperative care; as with the randomized subjects, self-reported outcomes were statistically better in the surgical group at 2 years.

REFERENCES

1. Bush K, Cowan N, Katz DE, Gishen P. The natural history of sciatica associated with disc pathology: A prospective study with clinical and independent radiologic follow-up. *Spine*. 1992; 17(10): 1205–1212.
2. Atlas SJ, Keller RB, Wu YA, Deyo RA, Singer DE. Long-term outcomes of surgical and nonsurgical management of sciatica secondary to a lumbar disc herniation: 10-year results from the Maine lumbar spine study. *Spine*. 2005; 30(8): 927–935.
3. Weinstein JN, Tosteson TD, Lurie JD, et al. Surgical versus nonoperative treatment for lumbar disk herniation: The Spine Patient Outcomes Research Trial (SPORT): A randomized trial. *JAMA*. 2006; 296(20): 2441–2450.
4. Weinstein JN, Lurie JD, Tosteson TD, et al. Surgical versus non-operative treatment for lumbar disc herniation: Four-year results for the Spine Patient Outcomes Research Trial (SPORT). *Spine*. 2008; 33(25): 2789.
5. Weinstein JN, Tosteson TD, Lurie JD, et al. Surgical versus nonoperative treatment for lumbar disk herniation: The Spine Patient Outcomes Research Trial (SPORT) observational cohort. *JAMA*. 2006; 296(20): 2451–2459.

Radiculopathy and Myelopathy at Segments Adjacent to the Site of a Previous Anterior Cervical Arthrodesis*

Hilibrand AS, Carlson GD, Palumbo MA, et al. J Bone Joint Surg Am 81:519–528, 1999

Reviewed by Godefroy Hardy St-Pierre and Ken Thomas

Research Question/Objective Anterior cervical arthrodesis is believed to lead to an accelerated progression of adjacent segment degeneration. While providing excellent short-term results, the longevity of the procedure is brought into question via additional biomechanical stress at the unfused levels above and below. Further ambiguity arises with the lack of clear association between radiological degeneration postoperatively and symptomatic clinical disease attributable to the adjacent segment. Contrary to prior studies, Hilibrand et al. focused on symptomatic adjacent segment disease (ASD), rather than radiological, up to 10 years post–cervical arthrodesis. They determined the incidence and prevalence of this disease and explored potential causative factors.

Study Design A cohort study of patients who underwent anterior cervical arthrodesis by a single surgeon at a single institution.

Sample Size Three hundred seventy-four patients undergoing 409 procedures over 19 years (1972–1992)

Follow-Up One to 10 years. Median 4 years.

Inclusion/Exclusion Criteria Inclusion criteria are not explicitly cited in the article. Excluded were 9 patients that died within 6 months of the index procedure as well as patients with acute fracture or dislocation, or malignant neoplasm, or those scheduled for a concomitant posterior arthrodesis.

Intervention Anterior cervical arthrodesis via a modified Smith-Robinson technique. The procedure was performed at all levels with

---

* Hilibrand AS, Carlson GD, Palumbo MA, et al. Radiculopathy and myelopathy at segments adjacent to the site of a previous anterior cervical arthrodesis. *J Bone Joint Surg.* 1999; 81: 519–528.

attributable symptoms of either radiculopathy or myelopathy in 338 procedures. In another 71 procedures, a subtotal vertebrectomy and arthrodesis with strut grafting was performed for advanced spondylosis or congenital stenosis with spinal cord compression.

Results   Clinical ASD presented in 58 of the 409 procedures, representing an overall prevalence of 14.2%. New symptomatic ASD presented at a constant rate over the 10-year postoperative period at an average annual incidence of 2.9% per year. Kaplan-Meier analysis predicted a prevalence of 13.6% at 5 years and 25.6% at 10 years. Of the 55 patients with clinical ASD, 27 underwent reoperation at the adjacent segment. There were significant differences between the cervical levels with C5-C6 and C6-C7 being at highest risk of reoperation, while C2-C3 and T1-T2 were at the lowest risk. Those results seemed to correlate location of clinical ASD with the amount of motion in flexion/extension. Contrary to the authors' initial hypothesis, multilevel arthrodesis was found to be associated with a significantly lower prevalence of clinical ASD (OR 0.64 $p < 0.001$). Finally, preoperative radiological degeneration, not addressed at the time of the index surgery, was correlated with an earlier onset of clinical ASD.

The prevalence of clinical ASD in this study was much higher than previously reported, most likely secondary to the long duration of follow-up and the inclusion of both operative and nonoperative patients in the new clinical ASD group. The finding that multilevel arthrodesis imparted a lower risk of clinical ASD supports the hypothesis that clinical ASD is due to progression of existing cervical spondylosis, as opposed to excessive motion at unfused segments. This was consistent with their radiological analysis of initial degeneration and, if not addressed surgically, its correlation with earlier onset of clinical ASD. The authors finally advocated incorporating all degenerated segments in the construct to minimize reoperation.

Study Limitations   Despite being accounted for through sound statistical methodology, 10%–20% of patients were lost to follow-up each year, with the potential to greatly alter the results, including the steady rate of clinical ASD postoperatively. With the exception of multilevel versus single level, no further stratification or subgroup analysis was provided despite the heterogeneity of the procedures performed. Likewise, no information was provided as to which procedure was performed at which specific level. The radiological analysis was again similarly weakened by the use of three different modalities to assess the presence of degenerative changes with widely different sensitivities for such findings. Finally, the outcomes of patients without clinical ASD were not provided, thus preventing an answer as to whether the occurrence of clinical ASD influences overall outcome.

Relevant Studies   The authors opened an entirely new field of study by bringing the notion of adjacent segment disease to the forefront of the literature. Numerous reports[1,2] have confirmed their findings, the most important being that cervical clinical ASD was much more common than previously thought; despite initial skepticism,[3] the concept has been firmly established.[4–6]

Even with more widespread recognition of clinical ASD, the exact cause of adjacent segment disease remains unclear.[7] The initial report established that the natural history of cervical spondylolysis was the determining factor in the appearance of clinical ASD. Further studies suggested that the fusion itself might be a factor through increased biomechanical stress,[1–6] although this commonly held belief has at most indirect evidence.[7–9] Matsumoto et al.[9] compared the natural history of radiological changes over 10 years between asymptomatic volunteers to patients treated with cervical arthrodesis. Progression of degeneration was more rapid in the cervical arthrodesis group. To draw a conclusion that the arthrodesis caused accelerated degenerative changes is inherently flawed by selection bias, bias in that the cervical arthrodesis group may not have been the same at inception as they started out with symptomatic disease—this possibly being a surrogate for a propensity toward degenerative changes.

The recognition of clinical ASD has led to a search for preventative strategies such as the use of cervical total disk replacement (cTDR). This led to numerous randomized controlled trials comparing cTDR to cervical arthrodesis.[10–14] This new literature confirmed Hilibrand et al. findings with remarkably similar rate of ASD for cervical arthrodesis, with no reduction of clinical ASD for cTDR.[15–19] This failure to demonstrate any significant prevention of clinical ASD lends credence to the notion that this entity was linked to the progression of cervical spondylosis, as initially postulated by Hilibrand et al.

REFERENCES

1. Ishihara H, Kanamori M, Kawaguchi Y, et al. Adjacent segment disease after anterior cervical interbody fusion. *Spine J.* 2004; 4(6): 624–628.
2. Yue WM, Brodner W, Highland TR. Long-term results after anterior cervical discectomy and fusion with allograft and plating. *Spine.* 2005; 30(19): 2138–2144.
3. Moonsang S, Choi D. Adjacent segment disease after fusion for cervical spondylosis: Myth or reality? *Br J Neurosurg.* 2008; 22(2): 195–199.
4. Hilibrand AS, Robbins M. Adjacent segment degeneration and adjacent segment disease: The consequence of spinal fusion? *Spine J.* 2004; 4(6): S190–S194.
5. Lawrence BD, Hilibrand AS, Brodt ED, et al. Predicting the risk of adjacent pathology in the cervical spine: A systematic review. *Spine.* 2012; 22S: S52–S64.
6. Chung JY, Kim SK, Jung ST, et al. Clinical adjacent-segment pathology after anterior cervical discectomy and fusion: Results after a minimum of 10 years follow-up. *Spine J.* 2014; 14(10): 2290–2298.

7. Hegelson MD, Bevenino AJ, Hilibrand AS. Update on the evidence for adjacent segment degeneration and disease. *Spine J.* 2013; 13(3): 342–351.
8. Harrod CC, Hilibrand AS, Fischer DJ, et al. Adjacent segment pathology following cervical motion-sparing procedures or devices compared with fusion surgery: A systematic review. *Spine.* 2012; 37(22S): S96–S112.
9. Matsumoto M, Okada E, Watanabe K, et al. Anterior cervical decompression and fusion accelerates adjacent segment degeneration: Comparison with asymptomatic volunteers in a ten-year magnetic resonance imaging follow-up study. *Spine.* 2010; 35(1): 36–43.
10. Mummaneni PV, Burkus JK, Haid RW, et al. Clinical and radiographic analysis of cervical disc arthroplasty compared with allograft fusion: A randomized controlled clinical trial. *J Neurosurg Spine.* 2007; 6: 198–209.
11. Sasso RC, Smucker JD, Hacker RJ, et al. Artificial disc versus fusion: A prospective, randomized study with 2-year follow-up on 99 patients. *Spine.* 2007; 32: 2933–2940.
12. Coric D, Nunley PD, Guyer RD, et al. Prospective, randomized, multicenter study of cervical arthroplasty: 269 patients from the Kineflex C artificial disc investigational device exemption study with a minimum 2-year follow-up. *J Neurosurg Spine.* 2011; 15: 348–358.
13. Delamarter RB, Zigler J. Five-year reoperation rates, cervical total disc replacement versus fusion, results of a prospective randomized clinical trial. *Spine.* 2013; 38: 711–717.
14. Bae HW, Kim KD, Nunley PD, et al. Comparison of clinical outcomes of 1- and 2-level total disc replacement: Four-year results from a prospective, randomized, controlled, multicenter IDE clinical trial. *Spine.* 2015; 40(11): 759–766.
15. Jawahar A, Cavanaugh DA, Kerr EJ, et al. Total disc arthroplasty does not affect the incidence of adjacent segment degeneration in cervical spine: Results of 93 patients in 3 prospective randomized clinical trials. *Spine J.* 2010; 10(12): 1043–1048.
16. Nunley PD, Jawahar A, Kerr EJ, et al. Factors affecting the incidence of symptomatic adjacent-level disease in cervical spine after total disc arthroplasty. *Spine.* 2012; 37(6): 445–451.
17. Verma K, Gandhi SD, Maltenfort M, et al. Rate of adjacent segment disease in cervical disc arthroplasty versus single-level fusion. *Spine.* 2013; 38(26): 2253–2257.
18. Boselie TFM, Willems PC, van Mameren H, et al. Arthroplasty versus fusion in single-level cervical degenerative disc disease. *Spine.* 2013; 38(17): E1096–E1107.
19. Nunley PD, Jawahar A, Cavanaugh DA, et al. Symptomatic adjacent segment disease after cervical total disc replacement: Re-examining the clinical and radiological evidence with established criteria. *Spine J.* 2013; 13: 5–12.

CHAPTER 23

Surgical versus Nonsurgical Treatment for Lumbar Degenerative Spondylolisthesis

Weinstein JN, Lurie JD, Tosteson TD, et al. N Engl J Med 356:2257–2270, 2007

Reviewed by Akshay A. Gupte and Ann M. Parr

Research Question/Objective   The optimal management strategy for patients with lumbar spinal stenosis and degenerative spondylolisthesis remains a challenge to the spinal neurosurgical community. The goal of the published study was to report 2-year outcomes in patients with degenerative spondylolisthesis who were treated either surgically or with nonsurgical conservative management.

Study Design   The three components of the Spine Patient Outcomes Research Trial (SPORT)[1-4] sought to comprehensively examine different and common treatment options used to manage patients with intervertebral disc herniation, lumbar spinal stenosis, and lumbar degenerative spondylolisthesis. SPORT was a 5-year multicenter (11 states, 13 medical centers), multispecialty (neurosurgery, orthopedic surgery) prospective study with one arm randomized and the other observational that allowed patients to choose their preferred therapy. Both arms had identical selection criteria and outcomes assessments.

Sample Size   Of 892 eligible patients, 607 were enrolled in the current study. Of the 304 patients enrolled in the randomization group, 252 patients had follow-up data at 2 years. Similarly, of the 303 in the observational group, 269 patients had follow-up data at 2 years.

Follow-Up   Primary and secondary outcome measures were collected at 6 weeks as well as at 3, 6, 12, and 24 (listed only in detail in Table 23.1) months after enrollment. Scores were adjusted for age, sex, work status, depression, osteoporosis, joint problems, duration of current

Table 23.1   Change Scores and Treatment Effects for Primary Outcomes at 2 Years Postoperatively in the Randomized and Observational Cohorts Combined, According to Treatment Received

Primary Outcomes	Nonsurgical Treatment ($n = 187$)	Surgery ($n = 324$)	Treatment Effect of Surgery (95% CI)[c]
SF-36 Bodily pain[a]	$11.7 + 1.5$	$29.9 + 1.2$	18.1 (14.5 to 21.7)
SF-36 Physical function[a]	$8.3 + 1.5$	$26.6 + 1.3$	18.3 (14.6 to 21.9)
Oswestry Disability Index[b]	$-7.5 + 1.2$	$-24.2 + 1.0$	-16.7 (-19.5 to -13.9)

Source: Modified from Table 3 of Weinstein JN, et al. *N Engl J Med.* 2007; 356, 2257–2270.
[a] The SF-36 scores range from 0 to 100, with lower scores indicating severe symptoms.
[b] The Oswestry Disability Index ranges from 0 to 100, with higher scores indicating severe symptoms.
[c] Global *p*-value based on a Wald test assessing all time points simultaneously is less than 0.001 for all measures.

symptoms, reflex deficit, number of moderate or severe stenotic levels, baseline scores (for the SF-36, Oswestry Disability Index, and Stenosis Bothersomeness Index), and the treatment center.

Inclusion Criteria

Symptoms	Neurogenic claudication or radicular leg pain >12 weeks
Signs	Neurologic signs
Imaging	Spinal stenosis on cross-sectional scans
	Degenerative spondylolisthesis on lateral standing radiographs

Exclusion Criteria

Spondylolysis and isthmic spondylolisthesis

Intervention or Treatment Received   The surgical intervention consisted of posterior decompressive laminectomy with or without single-level fusion (iliac crest bone grafting ± pedicle screw placement posteriorly). Nonsurgical treatment could include physical therapy, epidural steroid injections, nonsteroidal medications and opioid drugs, or a combination of any of these.

Results   After adjusting for baseline confounding factors and eliminating the crossover effect (as-treated analysis), the authors concluded that symptomatic patients (>12 weeks) with degenerative spondylolisthesis improved significantly after surgical intervention in terms of their pain, function, and satisfaction for up to 2 years (Table 23.1).

The study design allowed for crossover of patients from one group (nonsurgical) to the other (surgical treatment). Forty-nine percent of the nonsurgical treatment group in the randomization arm and 25% of the nonsurgical treatment group in the observational arm underwent surgery by the end of 2 years. The authors postulate that this nonadherence to treatment was the main reason they were not able to find any statistical difference in the intention-to-treat analysis in the primary outcomes between the treatment groups across all follow-up time periods. They therefore performed an as-treated analysis, which showed statistically significant results in favor of surgical intervention for all primary as well as secondary outcomes. They reported that these treatment effects remained robust across all follow-up time periods.

Study Limitations The substantial crossover rates observed in this study compromise the internal validity of the intention-to-treat analysis. The authors were able to counter this challenge through the presentation of the as-treated analysis; however, this may have introduced bias in terms of patients' preexisting ideas of the benefits of surgical versus nonsurgical interventions.

Another study limitation was the significant variation among nonsurgical treatment options offered (epidural steroid injections, opioid medications, nonsteroidal medications, and physical therapy), rendering it difficult to evaluate individual treatment effects of these conservative measures. The frequency of these nonsurgical subtreatments was different than what other research articles have reported. For example, the Maine Lumbar Spine Study[5] (MLSS) reported lower rates of epidural injections (18%) compared to SPORT (44%), making comparison between them difficult.[5,6] Similarly, the surgical techniques and extent of fusion also varied, and therefore direct comparisons between specific operative and nonoperative interventions were not possible.

Relevant Studies Since this study was published, further follow-up data has been made available.[2] At 4 years after surgery, the authors concluded that, compared with patients who were treated nonoperatively, patients who were treated surgically maintained substantially greater pain relief and improvement in function for 4 years.

In 2009, Chou et al.[7] reviewed the benefits of surgery on symptomatic spinal stenosis, herniated disc causing radiculopathy, and nonradicular back pain due to degenerative changes. They found a total of 17 trials looking at laminectomy with or without fusion in patients with spinal stenosis (± spondylolisthesis). Only 2 of these trials had $n > 100$. In this review they found a moderate benefit at 1–2 years of follow-up for surgical therapy compared to nonoperative conservative therapy.

In 2016, Zaina et al.[8] published a systematic review looking at five randomized controlled trials (SPORT included) comparing surgical versus nonsurgical treatment options for lumbar spinal stenosis. They concluded that these trials provide low-quality evidence and conflicting results about the effectiveness of surgery versus nonoperative interventions for lumbar stenosis. However, all the trials do provide consistent evidence that surgical treatments have higher complication rates compared to nonoperative therapies. This review did not specifically examine patients with lumbar degenerative spondylolisthesis in addition to spinal stenosis.

The American College of Surgeons National Surgical Quality Improvement Program (NSQIP) database is a nationwide database that includes demographics, perioperative 30-day follow-up data, and variables across academic and private hospitals. Golinvaux et al.[9] recently compared SPORT to the NSQIP data and found similar perioperative factors and complication rates, thereby supporting the generalizability of SPORT.

Although this article focused on surgical versus nonsurgical strategies of managing degenerative spondylolisthesis, spine surgeons have also struggled with determining whether laminectomy or laminectomy with fusion is superior in treating symptomatic patients with similar presentation. Most recently, in April 2016, Ghogawala et al.[10] compared standard laminectomy versus laminectomy with posterolateral instrumented fusion in adult patients who had stable grade I spondylolisthesis in the Spinal Laminectomy versus Instrumented Pedicle Screw (SLIP) trial. In this randomized controlled trial ($n = 66$), patients who underwent laminectomy with fusion were associated with a statistically and clinically significant greater increase in the SF-36 physical component summary score (higher scores indicating better quality of life) at 2, 3, and 4 years postoperatively. In the same publication, Försth et al.[11] reported their randomized clinical trial of 247 patients with one- or two-level lumbar stenosis, with or without spondylolisthesis, and found no clinical benefit at 2 years postoperatively between patients who underwent decompression surgery alone compared to those who also received fusion surgery. Therefore, despite evidence that surgical intervention is beneficial for lumbar spinal stenosis and spondylolisthesis, the issue of which surgical intervention is the most beneficial remains unresolved.

REFERENCES

1. Weinstein JN, Lurie JD, Tosteson TD, et al. Surgical versus nonoperative treatment for lumbar disk herniation: The Spine Patient Outcomes Research Trial (SPORT) observational cohort. *JAMA*. 2006; 296(20): 2451–2459.
2. Weinstein JN, Lurie JD, Tosteson TD, et al. Surgical compared with nonoperative treatment for lumbar degenerative spondylolisthesis: Four-year results in the Spine Patient Outcomes Research Trial (SPORT) randomized and observational cohorts. *J Bone Joint Surg Am*. 2009; 91(6): 1295–1304.
3. Weinstein JN, Tosteson TD, Lurie JD, et al. Surgical versus nonsurgical therapy for lumbar spinal stenosis. *N Engl J Med*. 2008; 358(8): 794–810.
4. Weinstein JN, Tosteson TD, Lurie JD, et al. Surgical versus nonoperative treatment for lumbar disk herniation: The Spine Patient Outcomes Research Trial (SPORT): A randomized trial. *JAMA*. 2006; 296(20): 2441–2450.
5. Atlas SJ, Deyo RA, Keller RB, et al. The Maine Lumbar Spine Study, Part III: 1-year outcomes of surgical and nonsurgical management of lumbar spinal stenosis. *Spine (Phila Pa 1976)*. 1996; 21(15): 1787–1794; discussion 1794–1795.
6. Atlas SJ, Delitto A. Spinal stenosis: Surgical versus nonsurgical treatment. *Clin Orthop Relat Res*. 2006; 443: 198–207.

7. Chou R, Baisden J, Carragee EJ, Resnick DK, Shaffer WO, Loeser JD. Surgery for low back pain: A review of the evidence for an American Pain Society clinical practice guideline. *Spine (Phila Pa 1976)*. 2009; 34(10): 1094–1109.

8. Zaina F, Tomkins-Lane C, Carragee E, Negrini S. Surgical versus non-surgical treatment for lumbar spinal stenosis. *Cochrane Database Syst Rev*. 2016; 1: CD010264.

9. Golinvaux NS, Basques BA, Bohl DD, Yacob A, Grauer JN. Comparison of 368 patients undergoing surgery for lumbar degenerative spondylolisthesis from the SPORT trial with 955 from the NSQIP database. *Spine (Phila Pa 1976)*. 2015; 40(5): 342–348.

10. Ghogawala Z, Dziura J, Butler WE, et al. Laminectomy plus fusion versus laminectomy alone for lumbar spondylolisthesis. *N Engl J Med*. 2016; 374(15): 1424–1434.

11. Försth P, Olafsson G, Carlsson T, et al. A randomized, controlled trial of fusion surgery for lumbar spinal stenosis. *N Engl J Med*. 2016; 374(15): 1413–1423.

Surgical versus Nonsurgical Therapy for Lumbar Spinal Stenosis*

Weinstein JN, Lurie JD, Tosteson TD, et al. N Engl J Med 358:794–810, 2008

Reviewed by Chris Daly and Tony Goldschlager

Research Question/Objective Spinal stenosis is the most common indication for lumbar spine surgery in older adults.[1] The Spine Patient Outcomes Research Trial (SPORT) included the first randomized trial to compare surgical versus nonsurgical treatment of isolated lumbar canal stenosis without spondylolisthesis.

Study Design The lumbar stenosis component of SPORT was a multicenter trial consisting of a randomized controlled study and a concurrent observational cohort of patients who declined randomization. The authors posited that including patients who declined randomization would broaden the range of patients studied, thus increasing the generalizability of the trial findings.

Sample Size A total of 654 patients were enrolled, 289 in the randomized cohort and 365 in the observational cohort.

Follow-Up Follow-up time points were at 6 weeks, 3 months, 6 months, 1 year, and 2 years. Patients completed the Medical Outcomes Study 36-item Short-Form General Health Survey (SF-36) and the modified Oswestry Disability Index (ODI). Follow-up of the randomized cohort was 85% (255 of the 289 enrolled patients) at 12 months and 76% (221 patients) at 24 months. Follow-up of the combined cohorts at the 24-month time point was 83% (541 of the 654 enrolled patients).

Inclusion Criteria A minimum of 12 weeks of neurogenic claudication or radicular leg symptoms with confirmatory cross-sectional imaging demonstrating lumbar spinal stenosis at one or more levels and deemed to be a surgical candidate.

---

* Weinstein JN, Tosteson TD, Lurie JD, et al. Surgical versus nonsurgical therapy for lumbar spinal stenosis. *N Engl J Med.* 2008; 358(8): 794–810.

Exclusion Criteria   Degenerative spondylolisthesis and lumbar instability (defined radiologically as translation of more than 4 mm or 10 degrees of angular motion between flexion and extension on upright lateral radiographs).

Intervention or Treatment Received   The surgical protocol was standard posterior decompressive laminectomy. Six percent of patients underwent instrumented fusion. The nonsurgical protocol was "usual care" and recommended to include at least active physical therapy, education or counseling with home exercise instruction, and administration of nonsteroidal anti-inflammatory drugs, if tolerated.

Results   A total of 654 patients were enrolled, 289 in the randomized cohort and 365 in the observation cohort. Baseline characteristics were similar between the two cohorts. The observational cohort demonstrated more signs of nerve root tension and had stronger treatment preferences.

Primary outcomes were the modified Oswestry Disability Index (ODI), Short Form-36 (SF-36) bodily pain (BP), and physical function (PF) scales. Secondary outcomes consisted of low back pain, leg pain and stenosis bothersomeness indices, and assessments of patient satisfaction.

High rates of crossover/nonadherence were observed in the randomized cohort. Of those assigned to nonsurgical treatment, 43% underwent surgery within 2 years. Only 67% of patient assigned to surgery had undergone surgery at 2 years. The randomized cohort was analyzed on both intention-to-treat and as-treated bases, in combination with the observational cohort. On intention-to-treat analysis, a significant treatment effect favoring surgery was found on the SF-36 scale of bodily pain, 23.4 ± 2.3 for the surgical group compared with 15.6 ± 2.2 for the nonsurgical group, giving a treatment effect of 7.8 confidence interval (95% CI 1.5–14.1). No other primary outcome measure achieved statistical significance over the 2 years. The 2-year time point primary outcome measures can be seen in Table 24.1.

Analysis in an as-treated fashion, with pooling of the patients from the randomized and cohort studies, was also performed. Baseline analysis indicated

Table 24.1   Intention-to-Treat Analysis of Randomized Cohort at 2 Years

Outcome	Baseline Overall Mean	Randomized to Surgery	Randomized to Nonsurgical Treatment	Treatment Effect (95% CI)
No. of Patients Available for Follow-Up at 2 Years		108	113	
SF-36				
Bodily pain	31.9 ± 1.1	23.4 ± 2.3	15.6 ± 2.2	7.8 (1.5 to 14.1)[a]
Physical function	35.4 ± 1.4	17.1 ± 2.4	17.1 ± 2.3	0.1 (−6.4 to 6.5)
ODI	42.7 ± 1.1	-16.4 ± 1.9	-12.9 ± 1.8	−3.5 (−8.7 to 1.7)

[a]   Statistically significant treatment effect.

Table 24.2 As-Treated Analysis of Pooled Randomized and Observational Cohorts at 2 Years

Outcome	Baseline Overall Mean	As-Treated Surgery (mean change)	As-Treated Nonsurgical (mean change)	Treatment Effect (95% CI)
No. of Patients Available for Follow-Up at 2 Years		335	198	
SF-36				
Bodily pain	31.4 ± 0.6	26.9 ± 1.2	13.3 ± 1.4	13.6 (10.0 to 17.2)[a]
Physical function	34.9 ± 0.8	23.0 ± 1.3	11.8 ± 1.4	11.1 (7.6 to 14.7)[a]
ODI	43.2 ± 0.6	−20.5 ± 1.0	−9.3 ± 1.2	−11.2 (−14.1 to −8.3)[a]

[a] Statistically significant treatment effect.

that patients who underwent surgery were younger, more likely to be working, reported more pain, had lower levels of function, and had more psychological distress. The as-treated analysis revealed that the surgically treated group reported greater improvement in all measures compared with the nonsurgically treated patients, with statistically significant treatment effects evident at 6 weeks, reaching a maximum at 6 months and persisting until 2 years. The group treated nonsurgically reported moderate improvement over the 2 years. The results at the 2-year time point are detailed in Table 24.2.

Study Limitations   The SPORT lumbar spinal stenosis study was marked by high rates of nonadherence. As described above, 43% of those randomized to nonsurgical management underwent surgery, and only 67% those randomized to surgical management received surgery. This significantly reduced the power and value of intention-to-treat analysis.

Follow-up was a further limitation, with only 76% of patients from the randomized cohort available for follow-up at 24 months. The grouped cohort analysis is heavily influenced by patients who have chosen, rather than been randomized to, surgery. Of the 400 patients forming the surgical group, 308 elected to undergo surgery, rendering the study open to confounding influences and selection bias.

Relevant Studies   Four- and eight-year follow-up results of the Spine Patient Outcomes Research Trial Lumbar Spinal Stenosis Cohorts have been published.[2,3] The authors demonstrate persisting treatment benefits with regard to ODI, and SF-36 BP and PF for the observation cohort at 8 years following operative intervention. A smaller treatment benefit can be demonstrated for the randomized cohort when analyzed on an as-treated basis up to 4 years.

The Maine Lumbar Spine Study[4] and the Randomized Controlled Trial of Malmivaara et al.[5] also investigated surgical intervention for lumbar canal stenosis. The Maine Lumbar Spine Study,[4] a prospective cohort study of patients with lumbar spinal stenosis who underwent surgical decompression, demonstrated greater improvement than nonsurgically treated patients with regard to self-reported back and leg pain. Functional improvements observed at one year in the Maine lumbar spine surgical group and SPORT as-treated surgical group are similar (26.5 and 27.0, respectively, in the SF-36 PF score). Significantly smaller improvements in physical function were observed in the nonsurgically treated groups in the Maine study compared to those in the SPORT stenosis trial (1.0 and 10.5 in the SF-36 PF score at 1 year). On long-term follow-up at 8–10 years, surgically treated patients in the Maine series reported greater improvement in leg symptoms and back-related functional status than their nonsurgically treated counterparts.[6]

The randomized controlled trial of Malmivaara[5] compared patients with lumbar canal stenosis treated surgically and nonsurgically. The trial included patients with spondylolisthesis and demonstrated at 24 months an improvement in ODI following surgery of −12.8 points (versus −20.5 for the SPORT surgically treated cohort). ODI improvements observed in the nonsurgically treated patients at 24 months were −5.7 points in the Malimivaara et al.[5] cohort and −9.3 points for the SPORT cohort.

An additional recent randomized controlled trial comparing surgical management with physiotherapy (nonsurgical management) for lumbar spinal canal stenosis by Delitto et al.[7] is also confounded by significant (57%) crossover of the physiotherapy treatment arm to surgical treatment. The study reports no significant difference between surgical and physiotherapy management at 2 years with regard to the physical function component of the SF-36 and ODI. However, these findings must be interpreted in light of significant crossover.

REFERENCES

1. Deyo RA. Treatment of lumbar spinal stenosis: A balancing act. *Spine J.* 2010; 10(7): 625–627.
2. Weinstein JN, Tosteson TD, Lurie JD, et al. Surgical versus nonoperative treatment for lumbar spinal stenosis four-year results of the Spine Patient Outcomes Research Trial. *Spine.* 2010; 35(14): 1329–1338.
3. Lurie JD, Tosteson TD, Tosteson A, et al. Long-term outcomes of lumbar spinal stenosis: Eight-year results of the Spine Patient Outcomes Research Trial (SPORT). *Spine.* 2015; 40(2): 63–76.
4. Atlas SJ, Deyo RA, Keller RB, et al. The Maine Lumbar Spine Study, part II: 1-year outcomes of surgical and nonsurgical management of sciatica. *Spine.* 1996; 21(15): 1777–1786.
5. Malmivaara A, Slätis P, Heliövaara M, et al. Surgical or nonoperative treatment for lumbar spinal stenosis? A randomized controlled trial. *Spine.* 2007; 32(1): 1–8.
6. Atlas SJ, Keller RB, Wu YA, Deyo RA, Singer DE. Long-term outcomes of surgical and nonsurgical management of lumbar spinal stenosis: 8- to 10-year results from the Maine Lumbar Spine Study. *Spine.* 2005; 30(8): 936–943.
7. Delitto A, Piva SR, Moore CG, et al. Surgery versus nonsurgical treatment of lumbar spinal stenosis: A randomized trial. *Ann Intern Med.* 2015; 162(7): 465–473.

Surgical versus Nonoperative Treatment for Lumbar Disc Herniation: The Spine Patient Outcomes Research Trial (SPORT): A Randomized Trial*

Weinstein JN, Tosteson TD, Lurie JD, et al. JAMA 296(20):2441–2450, 2006

Reviewed by Christian Iorio-Morin and Nicolas Dea

Research Question/Objective   At the time of this study, lumbar discectomy was the most common surgical procedure performed in the United States for lumbar and leg pain. The effectiveness of the procedure was supported by a single prospective, randomized controlled trial for which the 10-year follow-up was published in 1983[1] as well as by multiple observational studies.[2] Considerable regional variation was observed in the rate of discectomies, highlighting differences in indications and perceived benefits among surgeons. The goal of this study was to provide reliable evidence surrounding the efficacy of lumbar discectomy compared to nonoperative treatment for lumbar intervertebral disc herniation.

Study Design   The Spine Patient Outcomes Research Trial (SPORT) was a large, multicenter prospective study encompassing three randomized controlled trials and three prospective observational cohorts comparing surgical and conservative management in lumbar disc herniation, spinal stenosis, and degenerative spondylolisthesis. The observational cohorts consisted of eligible patients who consented to the protocol follow-up schedule but refused randomization.

This article reports the 2-year results of the SPORT randomized controlled trial for disc herniation. The primary outcomes were changes from baseline in the bodily pain and physical function scales of the SF-36 Health Status Questionnaire and the Oswestry Disability Index (ODI). The secondary outcomes were measures of patient self-reported improvement, work status, and

---

* Weinstein JN, Tosteson TD, Lurie JD, Tosteson ANA, Hanscom B, Skinner JS, et al. Surgical vs nonoperative treatment for lumbar disk herniation: the Spine Patient Outcomes Research Trial (SPORT): a randomized trial. *JAMA.* 2006 Nov 22; 296(20): 2441–2450.

satisfaction with current symptoms and care. Symptom severity was measured using the Sciatica Bothersomeness Index.

Sample Size   A total of 501 eligible patients were enrolled from 13 centers in 11 U.S. states and randomized 1:1 between March 2000 and November 2004. Two hundred forty-five patients were assigned to receive surgery, while 256 were assigned to the nonoperative group.

Follow-Up   Follow-up questionnaires were completed at 6 weeks, 3 months, 6 months, 1 year, and 2 years following enrollment. Additional follow-ups were planned in the surgical group should the procedure be delayed to address potential biases resulting from differential follow-up timing between groups.

Inclusion/Exclusion Criteria   Patients were eligible if they had computed tomography (CT)- or magnetic resonance imaging (MRI)-proven lumbar disc herniation with corresponding radicular pain and clinical evidence of nerve root compression (positive straight leg raise test or femoral tension sign, asymmetrically depressed reflex, sensory or motor deficit in the appropriate distribution). All participants had to have undergone at least 6 weeks of nonoperative care and were 18 years or older.

Exclusion criteria included prior lumbar surgery, cauda equina syndrome, scoliosis greater than 15°, segmental instability (10° angular motion or 4-mm translation), vertebral fractures, spine infection or tumor, inflammatory spondyloarthropathy, pregnancy, comorbid conditions contraindicating surgery, or inability/unwillingness to have surgery within 6 months. Patients with multiple herniations were included if only one of the herniations was considered symptomatic.

Intervention   Patients were randomized to either operative or nonoperative treatment. Surgery consisted of a standard, midline, open discectomy, and nerve root decompression. Surgery was to be performed following enrollment, but a range for acceptable delay was not specified. Nonoperative treatment consisted of each center's "usual care" and included a minimum of active physical therapy, counseling with home exercise instruction, and nonsteroidal anti-inflammatory drugs if tolerated. The use of additional nonsurgical therapies was encouraged but not standardized.

Results   Of the 501 enrolled patients, 94% completed at least one follow-up. Baseline patient characteristics were similar between both groups, with a mean age of 42 years and the majority being white, employed males with posterolateral L5-S1 disk extrusions. Nonoperative treatment included education/counseling (93%), nonsteroidal anti-inflammatory drugs (61%), injections (56%), narcotics (46%), and physical therapy (44%). Surgical treatment was well tolerated, with a 5% rate of postoperative complications, the most common being dural tear (4%). Reoperation was performed in 4% of patients in the first year of follow-up, mostly for recurrent herniations at the same level.

Substantial nonadherence to treatment assignation was observed: Only 60% of the surgical group had undergone surgery after 2 years, while 45% of the nonoperative group had crossed over to receive surgery. Crossover patients were significantly different from adherent patients; patients who underwent surgery were younger, had a lower income, had worse baseline symptoms, had more baseline disability, and were more likely to rate their symptoms as getting worse at the time of enrollment.

In the intention-to-treat analysis, all measures of outcome showed strong improvement over time in both study arms. A plateau was usually reached by the 6-month follow-up, with further improvement being only marginal. There was no statistically significant benefit to surgery for all primary outcomes, including bodily pain, physical function, and ODI. Patients in the surgical arm did report decreased sciatica bothersomeness ($p = 0.003$) and a small increase in self-rated improvement ($p = 0.04$), while no difference was detected for work status, satisfaction with symptoms, and satisfaction with care.

The secondary as-treated analysis provided widely different results. For all primary outcomes and at all time points, a strong statistically significant benefit to surgery was identified after adjusting for potential confounders.

Study Limitations   The SPORT trial highlights the challenges of performing randomized controlled trials of surgical procedures.

The main limitation of SPORT resides in the significant nonadherence to randomized treatment. The strikingly high crossover rate creates a bias toward the null, which likely invalidates conclusions drawn from the intent-to-treat analysis and leads to an underestimation of the true effect of surgery. On the other hand, while the as-treated analysis provides a better assessment of the impact of the operative treatment itself, its results have to be interpreted with caution since half the patients chose their own treatment, treatment being essentially stratified according to disease severity. This latter analysis essentially became a high-quality prospective observational study subject to the very biases randomization was designed to eliminate. It seems clear, however, that both cohorts were associated with clinically significant improvement over time. Given the substantial crossover, most patients got the treatment they preferred, and most were satisfied with their outcome. This demonstrates that patients' preference should play a central role when treating lumbar disk herniation and that a shared decision-making process is key.

Second, there is considerable debate with regard to the ethics and logistics of performing sham surgeries, so that the controlled nature of the trial itself cannot completely exclude a placebo effect resulting from the surgical "experience."

Rather than a placebo procedure, the control group was a heterogeneous mix of various nonoperative interventions, acknowledging the fact that no standard conservative therapy existed. By not specifying a mandatory nonoperative treatment protocol, the authors aimed to keep the study generalizable at the expense of some internal validity.

Further limiting the external validity of the results was the self-selection of patients undergoing randomization. Of 1991 eligible subjects, 747 refused study participation; 743 refused randomization and were enrolled in the observational cohort; and only 501 (25%), fulfilling strict eligibility criteria, were randomized. Patients with more severe symptoms were three times more likely to decline randomization. Results from the observational study published simultaneously further showed that patients in the observational arm had substantially worse symptoms and chose to undergo surgery in 75% of cases.[3] The result was a highly selected, toned-down, randomized cohort from which the sickest patients were excluded. Because symptom severity had been shown to correlate with the benefit from surgery,[2] it is likely that the randomized SPORT cohort would underestimate the true benefit of surgery, regardless of crossover or any other bias. Conversely, this patient self-selection introduced a significant regression-to-the-mean bias in the as-treated analysis and the observational study, magnifying the treatment effect in the latter.

Relevant Studies   SPORT reception has been mixed, with multiple authors lavishing praise, while others harshly criticized the study for failing to conclusively answer its primary question.[4,5] Given its cost of $13.5 million, expectations were high that the trial would provide a definitive answer. The authors concluded that, because of the high crossover rate, no conclusion could be reached with regard to superiority or equivalence of surgery versus nonoperative management based on the intention-to-treat analysis. The long-term 4- and 8-year follow-ups showed persistent advantages in the as-treated analyses and no clinical deterioration over time in both groups.[6,7] These results supported the conclusions from the older Weber study[1] and the Maine Lumbar Spine Studies[2] that most patients improved over time regardless of surgery, but that improvement is quicker and slightly better at long-term follow-up in the surgical group. Later studies independently confirmed this trend,[8,9] which is now a widely accepted outcome. Another analysis of the SPORT data showed that increased symptoms duration is correlated with worse outcome, regardless of treatment strategy.[10] Last, an economic evaluation using the pooled data from the observational and randomized SPORT cohorts revealed that surgical treatment was moderately cost-effective when evaluated over a 2-year period, results being largely dependent on surgical costs.[11]

REFERENCES

1. Weber H. Lumbar disc herniation: A controlled, prospective study with ten years of observation. *Spine*. 1983; 8(2): 131–140.
2. Atlas SJ, Deyo RA, Keller RB, et al. The Maine Lumbar Spine Study, part II: 1-year outcomes of surgical and nonsurgical management of sciatica. *Spine*. 1996; 21(15): 1777–1786.
3. Weinstein JN, Lurie JD, Tosteson TD, et al. Surgical versus nonoperative treatment for lumbar disk herniation: The Spine Patient Outcomes Research Trial (SPORT) observational cohort. *JAMA*. 2006; 296(20): 2451–2459.
4. McCormick PC. The Spine Patient Outcomes Research Trial results for lumbar disc herniation: A critical review. *J Neurosurg Spine*. 2007; 6(6): 513–520.
5. Angevine PD, McCormick PC. Inference and validity in the SPORT herniated lumbar disc randomized clinical trial. *Spine J*. 2007; 7(4): 387–391.
6. Weinstein JN, Lurie JD, Tosteson TD, et al. Surgical versus nonoperative treatment for lumbar disc herniation: Four-year results for the Spine Patient Outcomes Research Trial (SPORT). *Spine*. 2008; 33(25): 2789–2800.
7. Lurie JD, Tosteson TD, Tosteson ANA, et al. Surgical versus nonoperative treatment for lumbar disc herniation: Eight-year results for the Spine Patient Outcomes Research Trial. *Spine*. 2014; 39(1): 3–16.
8. Osterman H, Seitsalo S, Karppinen J, Malmivaara A. Effectiveness of microdiscectomy for lumbar disc herniation: A randomized controlled trial with 2 years of follow-up. *Spine*. 2006; 31(21): 2409–2414.
9. Peul WC, van Houwelingen HC, van den Hout WB, et al. Surgery versus prolonged conservative treatment for sciatica. *N Engl J Med*. 2007; 356(22): 2245–2256.
10. Rihn JA, Hilibrand AS, Radcliff K, et al. Duration of symptoms resulting from lumbar disc herniation: Effect on treatment outcomes: Analysis of the Spine Patient Outcomes Research Trial (SPORT). *J Bone Joint Surg Am*. 2011; 93(20): 1906–1914.
11. Tosteson ANA, Skinner JS, Tosteson TD, et al. The cost effectiveness of surgical versus nonoperative treatment for lumbar disc herniation over two years: Evidence from the Spine Patient Outcomes Research Trial (SPORT). *Spine*. 2008; 33(19): 2108–2115.

2001 Volvo Award Winner in Clinical Studies: Lumbar Fusion versus Nonsurgical Treatment for Chronic Low Back Pain: A Multicenter Randomized Controlled Trial from the Swedish Lumbar Spine Study Group*

Fritzell P, Hagg O, Wessberg P, et al. Spine 26(23):2521–2532, 2001

Reviewed by Andrew B. Shaw, Daniel S. Ikeda, and H. Francis Farhadi

Research Question/Objective Lumbar fusion for the treatment of lower back pain remains controversial.[1] Seventy to eighty-five percent of the population experience lower back pain at some time in their lives. Back pain is the most common cause of activity limitation in people younger than 45.[2] The management of chronic low back pain has involved both conservative measures including analgesics, physiotherapy, injections, and surgery. The primary aim of this study was to determine if lumbar fusion could reduce pain and disability greater than nonsurgical treatment in patients with chronic low back pain. Pain, disability, global self-rating, and return to work were used as primary outcome measures.

Study Design This was a multicenter, randomized controlled study with 2-year follow-up performed by an independent observer comparing surgical versus nonsurgical management of low back pain. The observer used validated questionnaires.

Sample Size Three hundred ten patients were referred from primary care physicians to 19 orthopedic departments from 1992 to 1998 in Sweden. Sixteen patients were excluded, leaving 294 patients that were randomized.

* Fritzell P, Hagg O, Wessberg P, Nordwall A, Swedish Lumbar Spine Study G. 2001 Volvo Award Winner in Clinical Studies: Lumbar fusion versus nonsurgical treatment for chronic low back pain: A multicenter randomized controlled trial from the Swedish Lumbar Spine Study Group. *Spine.* Dec 1 2001; 26(23): 2521–2532; discussion 2532–2524.

Two hundred twenty-two were randomized to the surgical group, and 72 were included in the control group; 219 in the surgical group and 70 in the control group completed the study through 2 years of follow-up.

Follow-Up   Pain (Visual Analogue Scale (VAS) back and leg) as well as complications were documented at 6 months, 12 months, and 2 years. Baseline questionnaires including Oswestry Disability Index (ODI), Million Visual Analogue Score (MVAS), General Function Score (GFS), Zung Self-Rating Depression Scale, patient overall assessment, work status, and compensation were repeated at the final follow-up and assessed for statistical significance.

Inclusion/Exclusion Criteria   Twenty-five- to sixty-five-year-old patients of both sexes with severe chronic low back pain for at least 2 years were included. Back pain intensity had to be greater than leg pain and not include signs of nerve root compression. The treating surgeon was required to evaluate the patient based on history/symptomatology, physical exam, and imaging to interpret the pain as being derived from either L4-L5 or L5-S1. Patients must have been on sick leave for at least 1 year and failed conservative measures. They must have scored at least 7 of 10 points for 10 questions reflecting "Function and Working Disability." A score of 10 correlates with "severe pain, no function with total handicap, no working ability." Degenerative changes at L4-L5 and L5-S1 on X-ray, computed tomography (CT), and/or magnetic resonance imaging (MRI) were required. A herniated disk was allowed if there was no clinical evidence of nerve root compression. Other medical comorbidities were allowed when deemed appropriate by the treating surgeon. Patients with ongoing psychiatric illness were not allowed to participate. Patients who had a history of spine surgery were excluded except for those who underwent discectomies greater than 2 years prior with successful removal of the disk and without persistent nerve root symptoms. The presence of radiologic findings including spondylolisthesis, fractures, infection, neoplasm, and inflammatory processes precluded participation.

Employment status or ongoing litigation were not used to include/exclude patients.

Intervention   The primary aim of this study was to determine whether lumbar fusion could reduce pain and disability greater than nonsurgical treatment. The investigators thus established two groups, surgical and nonsurgical. The surgical group was treated by any one of 26 experienced spine surgeons. All cases utilized autologous bone from the iliac crest. The surgical group was further divided into three groups: in situ fusion with decortication but without posterolateral fusion (PLF), variable screw placement (VSP), or circumferential fusion (360°) with the use of iliac crest bone and interbody grafts placed through either posterior or anterior approaches. All patients were provided with corset braces postoperatively and underwent early mobilization. Only L4-L5 and L5-S1 levels were addressed.

The nonsurgical group involved treatment primarily with physical therapy, but other forms of treatment were allowed, including education, transcutaneous electrical nerve stimulation (TENS), acupuncture, injections, cognitive/functional training, and coping strategies. The treatment received could vary significantly, but all were within commonly used treatment paradigms.

Results A total of 310 patients were randomized between 1992 and 1998, but 16 were excluded, leaving 294 patients allocated to surgical treatment ($n = 222$) or nonsurgical treatment ($n = 72$). Follow-up was 98% at 2 years, with males comprising 49.5% and 48.6% of the surgical and nonsurgical groups, respectively. The average duration of chronic low back pain was 7.8 and 8.5 years in the surgery and nonsurgical groups, respectively. Fusions were performed in 211 out of 222 patients. Of these 211 patients, 122 were fused at a single level and 89 at two levels. No significant differences were present in demographic and clinical characteristics. At 2-year follow-up, back pain in the surgical group was reduced by 32.7% compared with 6.8% in the nonsurgical group. Greater improvement was seen in the first 6 months, with gradual worsening of pain over the 2-year follow-up. Outcomes were significantly improved in the surgical group compared to the nonsurgical group in all measures including the ODI, MVAS, GFS, and the Zung Self-Rating Depression scale. The ODI improved by 24.5% in the surgical group compared to 5.8%, the MVAS by 28.4% compared to 7.8%, the GFS improved by 30.5% compared to 4.4%, and the Zung scale by 20% compared to 7%. The patients also rated their outcomes as improvement ("much better or better") or no improvement ("unchanged or worse"), with 63% in the surgical group reporting improvement compared to 29% in the nonsurgical group. Of note, 75% of the patients in the surgical group reported they would go through surgery again knowing their 2-year outcomes compared with 53% in the nonsurgical group. Complication rates are essential considerations when considering surgery versus nonsurgical management; in this study, 17% of patients in the surgical group suffered an early complication, including infection, new pain/radiculopathy from a badly positioned hardware, cerebrospinal fluid (CSF) leak, deep vein thrombosis/pulmonary embolus (DVT/PE), and positioning-related nerve injuries.

Study Limitations Fritzell and colleagues demonstrated the ability to perform a rigorous, randomized controlled study evaluating surgical intervention for a challenging clinical problem. However, there were some important limitations to the study. First, the management employed in the nonsurgical arm was variable. Rehabilitation services were noted to be a main component, but other adjuncts utilized were variable and unknown. In addition, patients may have undergone previous conservative measures without improvement, resulting in their presentation to a spine surgeon. Further, the generalizability of this study to the general population is limited given that the levels evaluated were isolated to L4-L5 and L5-S1 and that no radicular component was allowed. Degenerative disc disease is often noted at more than one or two levels, which is an exclusion for this trial. Curiously, patients that reported themselves as "unchanged or worse" expressed a feeling of satisfaction. This reflects the challenge in trial design and execution given that the experience of pain is often both subjective and affective. The increased attention and medical care may have independently resulted in improvement even if surgery itself was not beneficial. At 2-year follow-up, there remained considerable pain and disability with only 29% in the surgical group reporting to be "much better." It is important to remember that the procedure was not curative but rather reduced pain and disability.

Relevant Studies   This study addresses an important question regarding surgical intervention versus continued nonsurgical management for disabling chronic lower back pain. However, controversy remains on the ideal treatment for back pain given the high rates of fusion surgeries performed in the United States.[1] The Swedish Lumbar Spine Study Group included several different techniques for surgical intervention, including posterolateral fusion, fusion with pedicle screws, and interbody fusion with pedicle screw placement. The comparison between these techniques was published in a separate subgroup analysis where all three surgeries resulted in similar improvements in pain and disability but varied greatly in early complication rates; circumferential fusion had the highest at 31%.[3] However, successful fusion rates were also highest in the circumferential fusion group, with 91% fusion compared to 72% fusion in the posterolateral fusion group. The Study Group also looked at overall complication rates when comparing the three surgical procedures. They found no difference in clinical outcomes, but the total complication rates at 2-years for the PLF, VSP, and 360° groups were 12%, 22%, and 40%, respectively. The need for revision surgery was 6% for the PLF, 22% for the VSP, and 17% for the circumferential group.[4] The authors emphasized the need for further study and consensus regarding best practices given similar clinical outcomes regardless of the procedure selected.

Cognitive therapy has been shown to provide sustained improvement in back pain (at 12 months), both self-reported and observational.[5] Brox and colleagues performed a single blind randomized study comparing the effectiveness of lumbar instrumented fusion to cognitive intervention and exercise in patients with chronic low back pain and disk degeneration.[6] Sixty-four patients with low back pain and degenerative disease at L4-L5 and L5-S1 were evaluated for longer than one year and were randomized to instrumented fusion with PT versus cognitive therapies with exercise. The study found equal improvement in low back pain and disability between the two treatment arms. These findings further support the importance of the affective component of the pain experience.

Alternatives to spinal surgery for chronic low back pain include neuromodulation with spinal cord stimulation. Al Kaisy and colleagues performed a prospective, multicenter observational study to evaluate the long-term benefit of high frequency stimulation (10 kHz) for the treatment of chronic intractable back and leg pain.[7] This study showed significant improvement in back and leg pain from a baseline VAS of 8.4 down to 3.3 (back) and 5.4 down to 2.3 (leg) after 24 months of therapy. In addition, there were significant reductions in opioid use and sleep disturbances as well as ODI improvements. Burst spinal cord stimulation as an alternative to tonic stimulation has been shown to be effective in reducing both back and leg symptoms and may provide an alternative programming option for neuromodulators.[8]

The Swedish Spine Study Group also analyzed health outcomes and cost effectiveness of surgery. Further randomized trials are necessary to determine best practices, both surgical and nonsurgical, for the treatment of patients with chronic back pain.

REFERENCES

1. Deyo RA, Nachemson A, Mirza SK. Spinal-fusion surgery: The case for restraint. *N Engl J Med.* 2004; 350(7): 722–726.
2. Andersson GB. Epidemiological features of chronic low-back pain. *Lancet.* 1999; 354(9178): 581–585.
3. Fritzell P, Hagg O, Wessberg P, Nordwall A. Swedish Lumbar Spine Study Group. Chronic low back pain and fusion: A comparison of three surgical techniques: A prospective multicenter randomized study from the Swedish Lumbar Spine Study Group. *Spine.* 2002; 27(11): 1131–1141.
4. Fritzell P, Hagg O, Nordwall A. Swedish Lumbar Spine Study Group. Complications in lumbar fusion surgery for chronic low back pain: Comparison of three surgical techniques used in a prospective randomized study: A report from the Swedish Lumbar Spine Study Group. *Eur Spine J.* 2003; 12(2): 178–189.
5. Turner JA, Jensen MP. Efficacy of cognitive therapy for chronic low back pain. *Pain.* 1993; 52(2): 169–177.
6. Brox JI, Sorensen R, Friis A, et al. Randomized clinical trial of lumbar instrumented fusion and cognitive intervention and exercises in patients with chronic low back pain and disc degeneration. *Spine.* 2003; 28(17): 1913–1921.
7. Al-Kaisy A, Van Buyten JP, Smet I, Palmisani S, Pang D, Smith T. Sustained effectiveness of 10 kHz high-frequency spinal cord stimulation for patients with chronic, low back pain: 24-month results of a prospective multicenter study. *Pain Med.* 2014; 15(3): 347–354.
8. De Ridder D, Plazier M, Kamerling N, Menovsky T, Vanneste S. Burst spinal cord stimulation for limb and back pain. *World Neurosurg.* 2013; 80(5): 642–649, e641.

CHAPTER 27

Cervical Spine Fusion in Rheumatoid Arthritis

Ranawat CS, O'Leary P, Pellicci P. J Bone Joint Surg Am 61(7):1003–1010, 1979

Reviewed by Andrew H. Milby and Harvey E. Smith

Research Question/Objective Involvement of the cervical spine is common in patients with moderate or severe rheumatoid arthritis. Pain and neurologic compromise may result from instability of the atlantoaxial or subaxial articulations, or from superior migration of the dens into the foramen magnum. The authors sought to classify these patterns based on their clinical presentations and radiographic characteristics, and to describe the associated outcomes following their operative interventions.

Study Design A retrospective review of patients with rheumatoid arthritis undergoing cervical spinal fusion from 1969 to 1976 was performed. Patients were classified as to their preoperative functional status using the American Rheumatism Association functional classification. A novel classification scheme was also applied, including grading of pain from 0 to 3 based on severity, and assessment of neurologic status in three classes, including a subdivision of the third class based on ambulatory status (Table 27.1). This classification scheme was applied preoperatively and postoperatively to assess ultimate clinical outcomes following intervention. Radiographs were analyzed for evidence of atlantoaxial instability as described by Martel,[1] and subaxial subluxation as described by White.[2] The authors also introduce a novel method of assessing superior migration of the dens based on visualization of the C1 and C2 vertebrae and describe normative data from a population of 26 patients with unaffected spines to determine a normal threshold value (Figure 27.1).

Sample Size Thirty-three patients met inclusion criteria, representing 0.7% of the clinical population treated at the authors' institution during the study period.

Follow-Up Thirty of thirty-three patients survived the initial postoperative period. Subsequent follow-up for these patients ranged from 1 to 8 years.

Inclusion/Exclusion Criteria All patients met American Rheumatism Association criteria for diagnosis of rheumatoid arthritis, and underwent

Table 27.1 Ranawat Classification of Pain and Neurologic Status in Rheumatoid Arthritis

Pain Score	
0	None
1	Mild (intermittent, requiring only aspirin analgesia)
2	Moderate (cervical collar required)
3	Severe (unrelieved by aspirin or cervical collar)
Neurologic Class	
I	No neural deficit
II	Subjective weakness with hyperreflexia and dysesthesia
IIIA	Objective weakness and long-tract signs, but preserved ambulatory status
IIIB	Quadriparetic and nonambulatory

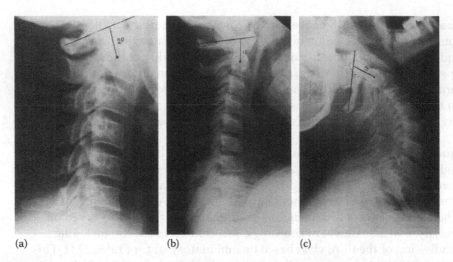

(a)   (b)   (c)

Figure 27.1 Ranawat technique for measurement of superior migration of the dens: (a) The diameter of the ring of the first cervical vertebra and the distance from the center of the pedicle of the second cervical vertebra to this diameter are determined. (b, c) The measurement of superior migration does not alter when the spine is in flexion or extension.

cervical spinal fusion during the study period for the indications of intractable pain and/or neurologic compromise in the setting of the three categories of radiographic findings described above. The three patients that died in the immediate postoperative period were excluded from statistical analysis.

Intervention or Treatment Received   Patients underwent the following surgical interventions based on their underlying pathology:

1. Anterior cervical fusion
2. Posterior Gallie fusion of C1 and C2 for atlantoaxial subluxation
3. Posterior fusion of occiput to C2 or C3 for superior migration of the dens

4. Long posterior fusion from occiput or upper cervical spine to lower subaxial cervical spine, with spinous process wiring for above pathologies in combination with subaxial instability

The following interventions were also performed in the perioperative period:

1. Preoperative halo traction in 14 patients with neurologic deficits in order to effect reduction
2. Postoperative halo-cast immobilization in 13 patients with poor bone quality or with fusions to the occiput
3. Postoperative hard cervical collar immobilization in all patients (unless halo in place) for minimum 3 months postoperatively until fusion evident on lateral flexion-extension radiographs
4. Preoperative tracheostomy in five patients with quadriparesis

Results Of the five patients undergoing anterior procedures, all were reported to have unsatisfactory outcomes. One patient who fused successfully in the reduced position was noted to have mild improvement in symptoms and ambulatory status. The remaining patients all had collapse or frank dislocation of their grafts, and no improvement in pain or neurologic status.

Of the 25 patients undergoing posterior procedures, nine underwent fusions from the occiput to C2 or C3 for treatment of atlantoaxial subluxation and superior migration of the dens. Three of these patients died within 2 months of surgery due to myocardial infarction, aspiration pneumonia, and sepsis from decubitus ulcers. Improvement or complete relief of pain was noted in five patients. Another patient was noted to have initial improvement but sustained a fall 3 months postoperatively, resulting in subaxial instability and loss of ambulatory capacity despite subsequent posterior decompression and later anterior fusion, and died 9 months following the index procedure.

Six patients underwent long posterior fusions, from the occiput, C1, or C2 cranially, to the lower subaxial spine or T1 caudally. Two of these patients died within 2 years of surgery of pneumonia and fat emboli, while the others generally improved in terms of pain and functional status.

Thirteen patients underwent Gallie fusion of C1 and C2 for isolated atlantoaxial instability. Two died within 2 months postoperatively; two others died within 1 year; seven had improved pain relief; three did not improve; and one worsened, requiring a second operation for pseudarthrosis. This reoperation was noted to be successful, with complete pain relief upon achievement of fusion.

The authors offer a detailed description of complications following these complex procedures in a challenging patient population. In total, they report three deaths in the immediate postoperative period, and another six within 2 years postoperatively for an overall mortality of 27% within the study period. They note a 20% (5/25) rate of pseudarthrosis among patients with sufficient long-term follow-up. Difficulties with management of pressure sores, and pin tract drainage in patients with halo immobilization are also discussed. The authors generally conclude that anterior fusions were less successful than posterior procedures, that intraoperative construct stability seemed to correlate with achievement of successful fusion, and that relief of pain was more predictable than improvement in neurologic or functional status. They propose that the largely irreversible nature of the myelopathy observed in this population may prompt a more aggressive approach to surgical stabilization in the presence of radiographic instability.

Study Limitations   While replete with candid and uncompromising detail regarding outcomes and complications, this study is not without significant limitations as a result of its retrospective nature and relatively small sample size. The authors propose a logical treatment algorithm for surgical planning based on the location and type of underlying instability; however, no comparisons between groups are possible as a result of the numerous variations in clinical presentation and individualized surgical treatment. Without control or comparison groups, it is not possible to state statistically whether surgical treatment is superior to the natural history of the disease or to nonsurgical immobilization; however, given the well-accepted natural history of cervical myelopathy, a control group study would be inappropriate. Advanced imaging modalities have since allowed for more precise identification of sites of pathology and more nuanced surgical planning. Also, the evolution of spinal instrumentation techniques since this article's publication may now allow for greater intraoperative stability and facilitate more extensive concurrent decompression than what was possible with the authors' instrumentation options (e.g., with modern spinal instrumentation, there is a markedly decreased utilization of postoperative halo vest immobilization). Last, the widespread use of disease-modifying antirheumatic drugs has changed the paradigm of inflammatory arthritis treatment, and may also affect the prevalence and distribution of the spinal sequelae of rheumatoid arthritis.

Relevant Studies   The authors note that their results are largely consistent with previously published reports. With modern instrumentation, C1-C2 posterior fusion with autograft, via either Goel-Harms technique or Magerl transarticular screws, has emerged as the mainstay of treatment for isolated atlantoaxial instability. Fusion constructs extending to the occiput are typically reserved for the treatment of superior migration of the dens, or when it is necessary to perform a C1 laminectomy in the setting of upper cervical instability. Preoperative traction may be used to effect reduction; if neurologic symptoms improve with traction, in situ fusion may be performed, with the potential to spare levels when compared to more extensive decompression. However, it is important to recognize and address subaxial instability at the time of the index procedure for upper cervical instability/basilar invagination (combined instability). Failure to recognize and address subaxial spine pathology at the time of the index upper cervical spine procedure can result in rapid deterioration of the caudal levels. Reported outcomes, including successful fusion and maintenance or improvement of neurologic status, vary widely and are highly dependent on the patient's disease severity and functional status at the time of surgery.[3-8] In general, superior outcomes have been obtained following surgery early in the disease process prior to the onset of severe myelopathy.[3,4,6,7,9]

REFERENCES

1. Martel W. The occipito-atlanto-axial joints in rheumatoid arthritis and ankylosing spondylitis. *Am J Roentgenol.* 1961; 86: 223–240.
2. White AA, Johnson RM, Panjabi MM, Southwick W. Biomechanical analysis of clinical stability of the cervical spine. *Clin Orthop.* 1975; 109: 85–96.
3. Boden SD, Dodge LD, Bohlman HH, Rechtine GR. Rheumatoid arthritis of the cervical spine: A long-term analysis with predictors of paralysis and recovery. *J Bone Joint Surg Am.* 1993; 75: 1282–1297.
4. Clark CR, Goetz DD, Menezes AH. Arthrodesis of the cervical spine in rheumatoid arthritis. *J Bone Joint Surg Am.* 1989; 71: 381–392.
5. Haid RW, Subach BR, McLaughlin MR, Rodts GE, Wahlig JB. C1–C2 transarticular screw fixation for atlantoaxial instability: A 6-year experience. *Neurosurgery.* 2001; 49: 65–70.
6. Peppelman WC, Kraus DR, Donaldson WF, Agarwal A. Cervical spine surgery in rheumatoid arthritis: Improvement of neurologic deficit after cervical spine fusion. *Spine.* 1993; 18: 2375–2379.
7. Matsunaga S, Ijiri K, Koga H. Results of a longer than 10-year follow-up of patients with rheumatoid arthritis treated by occipitocervical fusion. *Spine.* 2000; 25: 1749–1753.
8. Nagaria J, Kelleher MO, McEvoy L, Edwards R, Kamel MH, Bolger C. C1–C2 Transarticular screw fixation for atlantoaxial instability due to rheumatoid arthritis: A seven-year analysis of outcome. *Spine.* 2009; 34: 2880–2885.
9. Neva MH, Myllykangas-Luosujarvi R, Kautiainen H, Kauppi M. Mortality associated with cervical spine disorders: A population-based study of 1666 patients with rheumatoid arthritis who died in Finland in 1989. *Rheumatology.* 2001; 40: 123–127.

CHAPTER 28

Efficacy and Safety of Surgical Decompression in Patients with Cervical Spondylotic Myelopathy: Results of the Arbeitsgemeinschaft für Osteosynthesefragen Spine North America Prospective Multicenter Study

Fehlings MG, Wilson JR, Kopjar B. J Bone Joint Surg Am 95-A(18):1651–1658, 2013

Reviewed by Ajit Jada, Roger Härtl, and Ali Baaj

Research Question/Objective Cervical spondylotic myelopathy (CSM) is the most common cause of myelopathy in adults over 55 and a common cause of nontraumatic spinal cord injury and dysfunction globally. The focus of the current study was to evaluate the impact of surgical decompression on patients with CSM and to measure patient outcomes after 1 year using the modified Japanese Orthopaedic Association (mJOA) Scale, Nurick grade, Neck Disability Index (NDI), and Short Form-36 version 2 (SF-36v2).

Study Design *Prospective Cohort Study.* Adult patients with symptomatic CSM and MRI evidence of spinal cord compression were enrolled at 12 North American centers from December 2005 to September 2007. Clinical assessment was performed preoperatively, with symptom severity measured using mJOA score, Nurick grade, NDI, and SF-36v2. The same measurements were performed at several time points up to 1 year postoperatively and compared to preoperative values with univariate and multivariable paired statistics. Missing follow-up scores were accounted for using a multiple-imputation procedure. Treatment related complication data was compiled as well.

Sample Size Two hundred seventy-eight patients were initially enrolled in the study, 17 withdrew, and 1 died of an unrelated cause prior to 12-month follow-up. Two hundred sixty patients were followed for 1 year: 85 (30.6%) had mild CSM (mJOA ≥14), 110 (39.6%) had moderate CSM (mJOA 12–14), and 83 (29.9%) had severe CSM preoperatively (mJOA < 12).

Follow-Up   One-year follow-up data were available for 222 (85.4%) of the 260 patients, including 71 (91%) of the 78 with mild myelopathy, 89 (84.8%) of the 105 with moderate myelopathy, and 62 (80.5%) of the 77 with severe myelopathy.

Inclusion/Exclusion Criteria   Inclusion criteria were age of 18 years or older, symptomatic CSM, cervical cord compression on MRI, no prior surgical treatment for myelopathy, and the absence of symptomatic lumbar stenosis. There were no restrictions on duration of symptoms or prior nonoperative management.

Intervention   Patients received surgical decompression of the cervical spinal cord combined with instrumented fusion. The method of decompression was determined by the attending surgeon and was either an anterior, posterior, or circumferential approach. The number of vertebral segments decompressed and fused were determined by the surgeon as well.

Results   Patient age at presentation differed significantly among the severity groups. The mean age at presentation was higher for patients with severe disease and decreased for patients with moderate and mild disease. As expected, preoperative outcomes were progressively more favorable, from severe to moderate to mild disease. Also, the number of vertebral levels decompressed differed significantly among the groups, with more extensive decompressions performed in patients with severe disease compared to those with mild or moderate disease. There were no differences among the severity groups with respect to sex, smoking status, and preoperative duration of symptoms.

The authors found that overall the mJOA scores, Nurick grade, and NDI score improved significantly, from baseline to 1 year postoperatively, across all severity groups. Furthermore, significant improvements in health-related quality of life were observed for 9 of the 10 components of SF-36v2. Patients with mild disease preoperatively experienced the smallest improvement in the mJOA score and those with severe disease experienced the largest improvement.

Fifty-two patients (18.7%) had a total of 78 postoperative complications by 1-year follow-up. The complication rate did not differ among severity groups, and the most common complication was dysphagia in the early postoperative setting in 3.6% of patients, superficial infection constituted 2.9% of patients, and 6 patients (2.2%) required revision surgery. Indications for revision surgery included neck hematoma, deep wound infection, and graft malposition. Three patients had worsening myelopathy immediate postop; two of the three improved to baseline at 1-year follow-up.

Study Limitations The study was a prospective cohort without randomization. The authors mention that, from an ethical standpoint, not to operate on patients with myelopathy would not be feasible. Also, from a logistical standpoint, if a randomized controlled trial were implemented, the crossover rate from the nonoperative arm to the operative arm would undermine the randomized study design. Additionally, there was a 15% attrition rate at 1-year follow-up. Finally, the operations performed did not have a standardized surgical protocol and were performed by different surgeons at 12 institutions.

Relevant Studies As an adjunct to the current study, Dr. Fehlings's group published another prospective study analyzing predictors of surgical outcome in patients undergoing surgery for CSM.[1] The authors studied 757 patients treated surgically for CSM and identified those at 1-year follow-up who achieved an mJOA score of >16 and those who did not (mJOA < 16). The authors found that, based on univariate analyses, the probability of achieving a score of >16 decreased with the presence of certain symptoms, including gait dysfunction, certain clinical signs such as lower limb spasticity, positive smoking status, higher comorbidity score, more severe preoperative myelopathy, and older age. Patients were more likely to achieve an mJOA score of >16 if they were younger, had milder preoperative myelopathy, were nonsmokers, had fewer and less severe comorbidities, lacked gait impairment, and had shorter symptom duration.

Another review by the same group using the AO Spine CSM–International and North American data studied the comparison of outcomes of surgical treatment for ossification of the posterior longitudinal ligament (OPLL) versus other forms of degenerative cervical myelopathy (DCM).[2] The authors found that patients who underwent surgical decompression for treatment of OPLL experienced comparable outcomes to those seen in patients undergoing decompression for CSM. However, patients with OPLL were at a higher risk of perioperative complications compared to CSM patients.

Last, the authors also studied clinical and surgical predictors of complications following surgery for the treatment of CSM using the AO Spine CSM–International and North American data.[3] Of the 479 patients undergoing surgery for CSM, 78 patients experienced 89 perioperative complications. The univariate analysis revealed the major clinical risk factors were OPLL, number of comorbidities, comorbidity score, diabetes mellitus, and coexisting gastrointestinal and cardiovascular disorders. Those patients undergoing a two-stage surgery and those with longer operative durations also had a greater risk of perioperative complications. These findings were corroborated in a systematic review of the literature studying clinical and surgical predictors of complications following surgery for DCM.[4] The review also suggested that older patients are at a higher risk of perioperative complications, and longer operative duration and two-stage surgery are predictive of perioperative complications as well.

REFERENCES

1. Tetreault L, Kopjar B, Côté P, Arnold P, Fehlings MG. A clinical prediction rule for functional outcomes in patients undergoing surgery for degenerative cervical myelopathy: Analysis of an international prospective multicenter data set of 757 subjects. *J Bone Joint Surg Am.* 2015; 97(24): 2038–2046.
2. Nakashima H, Tetreault L, Nagoshi N, et al. Comparison of outcomes of surgical treatment for ossification of the posterior longitudinal ligament versus other forms of degenerative cervical myelopathy: Results from the prospective, multicenter AO Spine CSM–International Study of 479 patients. *J Bone Joint Surg Am.* 2016; 98(5): 370–378.
3. Tetreault L, et al. Clinical and surgical predictors of complications following surgery for the treatment of cervical spondylotic myelopathy: Results from the multicenter, prospective AO Spine International Study of 479 patients. *Neurosurgery.* 2016; 79(1): 33–44.
4. Tetreault L, Ibrahim A, Côté P, Singh A, Fehlings MG. A systematic review of clinical and surgical predictors of complications following surgery for degenerative cervical myelopathy. *J Neurosurg Spine.* 2016; 24(1): 77–99.

CHAPTER 29

Radiographic and Pathologic Features of Spinal Involvement in Diffuse Idiopathic Skeletal Hyperostosis*

Resnick D, Niwayama G. Radiology 119(3):559–568, 1976

Reviewed by Tyler Kreitz and Mark Kurd

Research Question/Objective   In this second of a two-part study by Resnick et al., the spinal radiographic and pathologic features of diffuse idiopathic skeletal hyperostosis (DISH) are described. Resnick et al. created the term DISH, previously labeled Forestier's disease, in an earlier manuscript describing the extraspinal manifestations of the disease.[1] This is the first study establishing diagnostic criteria for DISH, differentiating it from similar hyperostotic spine pathologies, for example, ankylosing spondylitis (AS) and intervertebral osteochondrosis or degenerative disc disease.

Study Design   Spinal radiographic and pathologic features of DISH were described. Cervical, thoracic, and lumbar radiographs of patients identified with patterns consistent with the disease were reviewed. Gross and microscopic pathology findings were described from dissection of cadaveric spines in patients with and without radiographic findings consistent with the disease.

Sample Size   The study included cervical, thoracic, and lumbar radiographs of 100 patients with findings consistent with DISH. Thoracic and lumbar vertebral column from 215 cadavers were chosen at random during postmortem examination. All radiographs and cadavers were collected from a single Veterans Affairs (VA) hospital.

Follow-Up   Not applicable.

---

* Resnick D, Niwayama G. Radiographic and pathologic features of spinal involvement in diffuse idiopathic skeletal hyperostosis (DISH). *Radiology*. 1976; 119(3): 559–568. doi:10.1148/119.3.559.

Inclusion/Exclusion Criteria   Radiograph inclusion criteria were based on findings from previous investigation of patients with advanced DISH, as no exact definition had been previously described. Criteria included (a) presence of "flowing" calcification along the anterolateral aspects of at least four contiguous vertebrae, (b) relative preservation of disc height in involved areas and the absence of extensive radiographic changes of "degenerative" disc disease, and (c) absence of apophyseal or sacroiliac ankylosis. Cadaver specimens were chosen at random from postmortem examinations.

Intervention   Not applicable.

Results   Of the 100 patients used in radiographic analysis, the mean age was 68 years (range of 49–88 years) and 96 were male, reflecting the VA population. The most common radiographic abnormalities were found in the thoracic spine (96%), specifically the seventh to tenth thoracic vertebrae. They describe a consistent pattern of flowing ossification along the anterolateral aspect of the vertebral bodies, between 1 and 20 mm thick, with underlying linear radiolucency separating ossification from vertebrae. An asymmetric pattern and predilection for the right side of the thoracic spine was seen. An overall "bumpy" appearance results from increased and more anterior deposition across disc spaces between involved vertebrae. Abnormalities were noted in 93% of available lumbar spine radiographs. Lumbar abnormalities were thick, up to 20 mm, and most commonly occurred along the third lumbar vertebrae. Cervical abnormalities were less frequent, occurring in 78% of radiographs. Cervical abnormalities also demonstrated flowing anterior ossification between 11 and 22 mm thick, occurring most commonly on the fifth and sixth cervical vertebrae. Progression of ossification was seen in all spine segments, beginning at the anterior vertebral body and gradually elongating across adjacent disc spaces. In advanced cases, underlying linear radiolucency disappeared with merging of anterior ossification and underlying sclerotic vertebral body. This pattern resulted in segmental ankylosis most commonly in the thoracic spine.

Twenty-five of the 215 cadavers examined (12%) demonstrated findings consistent with DISH. All 25 were male with an average age at death of 75 years (range 46–94 years). Age and cause of death were consistent with the cadavers not demonstrating DISH. Radiographic and pathologic examination of the spine was performed on all 25 cadavers. Calcification and ossification was seen primarily in the anterior longitudinal ligament (ALL), with predominance for the right side of the ALL. Disc space is preserved during early stages. As ossification of the ALL progresses, it extends across the anterior disc space, coalescing with a hypervascular and inflamed outer fibers of the annulus fibrosis. This extension coincides with merging of ossified ALL with sclerotic anterior vertebrae, resulting in the anterior flowing appearance on radiographs.

The results of radiographic and pathologic examination allowed for differentiation between DISH and similar pathologies, such as ankylosing spondylitis (AS), degenerative disc disease. DISH is most commonly seen in older patients (>50 years), most commonly affects the thoracic spine, and is characterized by flowing anterior ossification due to large nonmarginal osteophytes with preservation of intervertebral disc space, and apophyseal and sacroiliac joints. Modification of inclusion criteria from this study formed the initial diagnostic criteria for DISH: (1) "flowing" anterior ossification over four contiguous vertebrae, (2) relative preservation of intervertebral disc height, and (3) absence of apophyseal or sacroiliac joint changes.

Study Limitations   This retrospective-observational radiographic and pathologic examination evaluated a disease entity, DISH, which prior to this study lacked definitive diagnostic criteria. Selection of radiographs was based on previously reported patterns of ossification that differed from known pathologies, such as ankylosing spondylitis and degenerative disc disease. This study was performed at a single VA hospital and is limited by the demographics of that institution. In addition, there was no description of clinical manifestations associated with DISH, which in the context of the cervical spine, can often present with symptoms of progressive dysphagia.

Relevant Studies   Prior to this study, several terms had been used to describe the pattern of ossification seen in DISH. Oppenheimer first described this entity as *spondylitis ossificans ligamentosa* in 1942, based on radiographic ossification of spinal ligaments in the absence of intervertebral disc or apophyseal involvement.[2] It was proposed that spine immobility resulted in ossification of adjacent connective tissues.[2,3] Over time, the terms *spondylitis hyperostotica,*[4] *physiologic vertebral ligamentous calcification,*[5] and *generalized juxta-articular ossification of ligaments of the vertebral column*[6] would be used to describe this pattern. In 1971, Forestier et al. described ossification of the ALL predominantly in the thoracolumbar region, with associated extraspinal manifestations in the radiographic and pathologic evaluation of 245 patients.[7] These previous studies described similar findings: anterior spinal ossification, most commonly in the thoracic spine of older males.

Since their proposal in this study, the diagnostic criteria for DISH have remained consistent, with minor exceptions. The upper third ligamentous portion of the sacroiliac joint may demonstrate sclerosis and narrowing in patients with DISH.[8] The lower synovial portion remains intact, unlike the ankylosis seen in AS. This differentiation may be made by CT evaluation.[9] In 1978, Resnick et al. published a subsequent evaluation of cervical spine radiographs in patients with DISH demonstrating ossification of the posterior longitudinal ligament (PLL) in addition to the ALL. Among the 74 cervical radiographs evaluated, half demonstrated some degree of PLL ossification, with four demonstrating extensive

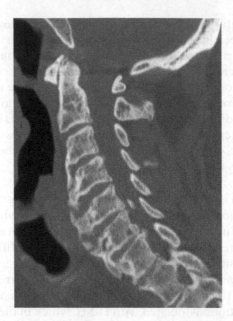

Figure 29.1 A midsagittal CT image of the cervical spine in a patient with diffuse idiopathic skeletal hyperostosis (DISH). Demonstrates anterior nonmarginal syndesmophytes from the third to seventh cervical vertebrae. This pattern is consistent with DISH.

calcification.[10] This finding may result in spinal stenosis. Predilection for right-sided ALL ossification likely results from influence of the pulsating thoracic aorta, as the opposite pattern is seen in situs inversus.[11] The etiology of DISH is still unknown, though there may be an association with insulin resistance and metabolic syndrome.[12] Previously DISH was considered a radiographic finding with limited clinical significance. Recent evidence suggests spinal manifestations of DISH may result in pain and functional limitations as well as dysphagia.[13] Those patients with severe manifestations of DISH may demonstrate spine immobility and postural deformity seen in advanced AS.[14]

This study defined DISH as an independent hyperostotic disease of the spine. It provided the initial diagnostic criteria for spinal manifestations seen in DISH (Figure 29.1). These criteria have remained consistent over time.

REFERENCES

1. Resnick D, Shaul SR, Robins JM. Diffuse idiopathic skeletal hyperostosis (DISH): Forestier's disease with extraspinal manifestations. *Radiology*. 1975; 115(3): 513–524, doi:10.1148/15.3.513.
2. Oppenheimer A. Calcification and ossification of vertebral ligaments (spondylitis ossificans ligamentosa): Roentgen study of pathogenesis and clinical significance. *Radiology*. 1942; 38: 160–173.

3. Leriche R, Policard A. Les problemas de la physiologie normale et pathologique de l'os. Paris: Masson Cie, 1926.
4. Ott V. Uber die Spondylosis hyperostotica. *Schweiz Med Wochenschr.* 1953; 83: 790–799.
5. Smith CF, Pugh DG, Polley HF. Physiologic vertebral ligamentous calcification: An aging process. *Am J Roentgenol Radium Ther Nucl Med.* 1955; 74(6): 1049–1058.
6. Sutro CJ, Ehrlich DE, Witten M. Generalized juxta-articular ossification of ligaments of the vertebral column and of the ligamentous and tendinous tissues of the extremities (also known as Bechterew's disease, osteophytosis and spondylosis deformans). *Bull Hosp Joint Dis.* 1956; 17(2): 343–357.
7. Forestier J, Lagier R. Ankylosing hyperostosis of the spine. *Clin Orthop.* 1971; 74: 65–83.
8. Yagan R, Khan MA. Confusion of roentgenographic differential diagnosis between anky-losing hyperostosis (Forestier's disease) and ankylosing spondylitis. *Clin Rheumatol.* 1983; 2(3): 285–292.
9. Yagan R, Khan MA, Marmolya G. Role of abdominal CT, when available in patients' records, in the evaluation of degenerative changes of the sacroiliac joints. *Spine.* 1987; 12(10): 1046–1051.
10. Resnick D, Guerra JJ, Robinson CA, Vint VC. Association of diffuse idiopathic skeletal hyperostosis (DISH) and calcification and ossification of the posterior longitudinal liga-ment. *AJR Am J Roentgenol.* 1978; 131(6): 1049–1053, doi:10.2214/ajr.131.6.1049.
11. Bahrt KM, Nashel DJ, Haber G. Diffuse idiopathic skeletal hyperostosis in a patient with situs inversus. *Arthritis Rheum.* 1983; 26(6): 811–812.
12. Kiss C, Szilagyi M, Paksy A, Poor G. Risk factors for diffuse idiopathic skeletal hyperosto-sis: A case-control study. *Rheumatol Oxf Engl.* 2002; 41(1): 27–30.
13. Mata S, Fortin PR, Fitzcharles MA, et al. A controlled study of diffuse idiopathic skeletal hyperostosis: Clinical features and functional status. *Medicine (Baltimore).* 1997; 76(2): 104–117.
14. Olivieri I, D'Angelo S, Cutro MS, et al. Diffuse idiopathic skeletal hyperostosis may give the typical postural abnormalities of advanced ankylosing spondylitis. *Rheumatol Oxf Engl.* 2007; 46(11): 1709–1711, doi:10.1093/rheumatology/kem227.

CHAPTER 30

Degenerative Lumbar Spondylolisthesis with Spinal Stenosis: A Prospective, Randomized Study Comparing Decompressive Laminectomy and Arthrodesis with and without Spinal Instrumentation*

Fischgrund JS, MacKay M, Herkowitz HN, et al. Spine 22(24):2807–2812, 1997

Reviewed by Philip K. Louie and Howard S. An

Research Question/Objective   The role of arthrodesis and fixation in the surgical management of degenerative spondylolisthesis with spinal stenosis in the lumbar spine has been the topic of much research over the past several decades. Previous studies had demonstrated improved clinical outcomes if arthrodesis was performed with decompression at the level of listhesis. Subsequent studies advocating for the addition of spinal instrumentation to enhance arthrodesis showed improved fusion rates, but the effect on clinical outcome remained uncertain. The goal of this study was to determine whether the addition of pedicle screw instrumentation would improve the fusion rate and clinical outcome of patients undergoing posterolateral fusion after decompression for spinal stenosis in the setting of degenerative spondylolisthesis.

Study Design   This was a prospective randomized study that evaluated the impact of adding transpedicular fixation on patient outcomes in the surgical management of spinal stenosis with degenerative spondylolisthesis. Patients were randomized to one of two treatment

---

* Fischgrund JS, Mackay M, Herkowitz HN, Brower R, Montgomery DM, Kurz LT. 1997 Volvo Award winner in clinical studies. Degenerative lumbar spondylolisthesis with spinal stenosis: A prospective, randomized study comparing decompressive laminectomy and arthrodesis with and without spinal instrumentation. *Spine*. 1997; 22(24): 2807–2812.

groups (segmental transpedicular instrumented or noninstrumented) at the time the decision was made to proceed with surgery.

Sample Size   Seventy-six consecutive patients with symptomatic spinal stenosis associated with degenerative spondylolisthesis at a single institution.

Follow-Up   Sixty-eight of 76 patients (89.5%) were followed for 2 years postoperatively.

Inclusion/Exclusion Criteria   Patients were included in the study if they satisfied all of the following criteria: clinical diagnosis of degenerative spondylolisthesis and spinal stenosis, underwent a minimum of 3 months nonoperative treatment, radiographic evidence of single-level degenerative spondylolisthesis, magnetic resonance imaging (MRI)/computed tomographic (CT) myelogram evidence of spinal stenosis at the level of the listhesis. Patients were excluded if they had undergone prior lumbar spinal surgery.

Intervention   Decompressive laminectomy and single-level bilateral intertransverse process arthrodesis with or without transpedicular instrumentation.

Results   The operation was performed at L4-L5 in 69 patients, at L3-L4 in 6 patients, and at L5-S1 in 1 patient. Of the 68 consecutive patients with 2-year follow-up, 55 were women and 13 were men. Thirty-five patients were randomized to the instrumentation group, while 33 were randomized to the noninstrumented cohort. The clinical outcome was excellent (patient resumed unrestricted activity and had near complete relief of pain in the back, lower limbs, or both) or good (occasional discomfort in the back or lower limbs, necessitating occasional non-narcotic medication) in 76% of the patients in whom instrumentation was placed and 85% of those in whom no instrumentation was used ($p = 0.45$). In 82% of the instrumented cases, successful arthrodesis was observed. However, only 45% of the noninstrumented cases revealed arthrodesis at 2 years after surgery ($p = 0.0015$). Successful fusion was not predictive of successful clinical outcome ($p = 0.435$).

Preoperative angular motion, spondylolisthesis, and sagittal motion did not significantly contribute to pseudarthrosis. There were no new peripheral neurologic deficits observed after surgery in either group. Five patients underwent reoperation. Two patients (one in each group) required a decompressive laminectomy at an adjacent level. One patient had hardware removed due to persistent low back pain; solid fusion was observed. One patient in the noninstrumented group experienced low back pain in the setting of pseudarthrosis and subsequently underwent an instrumented fusion. One patient in the instrumented group experienced recurrent stenosis and pseudarthrosis developed, requiring a second decompression and instrumented arthrodesis.

Study Limitations Limitations were not directly addressed in this study; however, limitations do exist. The 2-year follow-up is relatively short and may not accurately capture the long-term differences among clinical outcomes in those with a successful fusion compared to those in which a pseudarthrosis was present. Although no clinical differences were observed at 2 years postoperatively, longer-term follow-up may be necessary to evaluate the role of successful fusion in the clinical outcomes. Historically, the methods of evaluating a fusion mass have varied in the literature. Using radiographs to determine fusion status has traditionally been difficult; the current study evaluated fusion mass on radiographs as critically as possible; however, this method may factor into the low reported fusion rate in noninstrumented cases, which is contrary to their high clinical success rate.

Relevant Studies Some surgeons have reported clinical success after decompression alone for spinal stenosis in the setting of degenerative spondylolisthesis.[1] In 1991, Herkowitz and Kurz[2] published a prospective, randomized control trial comparing the results of decompressive laminectomy alone versus decompressive laminectomy and posterolateral fusion in degenerative spondylolisthesis. This landmark study revealed that patients who underwent an arthrodesis with the decompression experienced significant improvements in clinical outcome compared to those that did not undergo arthrodesis. Similar findings were described in a meta-analysis of operative treatments in degenerative spondylolisthesis by Mardjetko et al.[3] Patients that underwent a concomitant arthrodesis at the time of decompression experienced significantly better clinical outcomes that those that did not receive a fusion. The successful rate of fusion with rigid pedicle fixation had been previously described in studies evaluating multiple degenerative spinal conditions.[4,5] The current series was the largest prospectively randomized study on the use of pedicle screws for one diagnosis. Although the fusion rates were markedly increased in the instrumented group, there was no significant difference in clinical outcome between the two groups despite the high percentage of pseudarthrosis present in the noninstrumented cohort. These results were in agreement with the landmark findings by Herkowitz and Kurz,[2] and were thought to be related to the development of a fibrous fusion that provided sufficient structural support to prevent progressive spondylolisthesis.

In an effort to determine the long-term influence of pseudarthrosis on the clinical outcomes, Kornblum et al.[6] identified 47 patients with single-level symptomatic spinal stenosis and spondylolisthesis from this study. They selected patients treated with decompression and bilateral posterior arthrodesis with autogenous bone graft, but no instrumentation, and followed them for 5–14 years (average follow-up of 8 years). Long-term clinical outcome was excellent or good in 86% of the patients with solid arthrodesis but in only 56% of patients who developed a pseudarthrosis ($p = 0.01$). Although the fibrous union may benefit the patients in the short term (as seen at 2 years postoperatively), long-term outcomes appear to deteriorate without a solid fusion mass intact.

Following these landmark studies, the standard teaching has been decompression and fusion for patients presenting with symptomatic degenerative spondylolisthesis; sometimes however, the patient may similarly benefit from decompression alone or motion-preserving alternatives. Satisfactory clinical outcomes have been achieved with an isolated decompression in selected patients, avoiding the additional risks and costs of instrumentation and spinal fusion.[7-9] Specifically, radiographic parameters have been proposed in which patients would likely benefit without fusion (with or without instrumentation).[7] Additionally, others have challenged the notion of arthrodesis and have proposed that stabilization, not necessarily spinal fusion, may be sufficient and may further avoid complications that result following a traditional fusion procedure. Thus, less invasive, motion-preserving alternatives have been introduced to provide neural decompression and stabilization. The Graf, Dynesys, and Coflex systems have all showed promising clinical outcomes with 2- to 5-year follow-up data similar to patients who have received fusions with or without instrumentation.[1,10,11] Although further long-term studies are necessary, it is evident that the treatment for spinal stenosis in the setting of degenerative spondylolisthesis must be individualized, taking into account diverse demographic, pre- and intraoperative findings, and presenting symptoms. An essential component of the surgical intervention may rest in the ability to classify instability within degenerative spondylolisthesis. However, there is no current, widely accepted algorithm designed to provide surgeons with a decision-making model that would allow them to tailor their surgical treatment to patients presenting with a variety of symptoms, radiographic findings, and observed pathology in the setting of degenerative spondylolisthesis.

REFERENCES

1. Booth KC, Bridwell KH, Eisenberg BA, Baldus CR, Lenke LG. Minimum 5-year results of degenerative spondylolisthesis treated with decompression and instrumented posterior fusion. *Spine*. 1999; 24(16): 1721–1727.
2. Herkowitz HN, Kurz LT. Degenerative lumbar spondylolisthesis with spinal stenosis: A prospective study comparing decompression with decompression and intertransverse process arthrodesis. *J Bone Joint Surg Am*. 1991; 73(6): 802–808.
3. Mardjetko SM, Connolly PJ, Shott S. Degenerative lumbar spondylolisthesis: A meta-analysis of literature 1970–1993. *Spine*. 1994; 19(20 Suppl): 2256S–2265S.
4. Bridwell KH, Sedgewick TA, O'Brien MF, Lenke LG, Baldus C. The role of fusion and instrumentation in the treatment of degenerative spondylolisthesis with spinal stenosis. *J Spinal Disord*. 1993; 6(6): 461–472.
5. Zdeblick TA. A prospective, randomized study of lumbar fusion: Preliminary results. *Spine*. 1993; 18(8): 983–991.

6. Kornblum MB, Fischgrund JS, Herkowitz HN, Abraham DA, Berkower DL, Ditkoff JS. Degenerative lumbar spondylolisthesis with spinal stenosis: A prospective long-term study comparing fusion and pseudarthrosis. *Spine*. 2004; 29(7): 726–733, discussion 733–734.
7. Blumenthal C, Curran J, Benzel EC, et al. Radiographic predictors of delayed instability following decompression without fusion for degenerative grade I lumbar spondylolisthesis. *J Neurosurg: Spine*. 2013; 18(4): 340–346, doi:10.3171/2013.1.SPINE12537.
8. Joaquim AF, Milano JB, Ghizoni E, Patel AA. Is there a role for decompression alone for treating symptomatic degenerative lumbar spondylolisthesis? A systematic review. *J Spinal Disord Tech*. 2015: 1, doi:10.1097/BSD.0000000000000357.
9. Kim S, Mortaz Hedjri S, Coyte PC, Rampersaud YR. Cost-utility of lumbar decompression with or without fusion for patients with symptomatic degenerative lumbar spondylolisthesis. *Spine J*. 2012; 12(1): 44–54. doi:10.1016/j.spinee.2011.10.004.
10. Davis R, Auerbach JD, Bae H, Errico TJ. Can low-grade spondylolisthesis be effectively treated by either coflex interlaminar stabilization or laminectomy and posterior spinal fusion? Two-year clinical and radiographic results from the randomized, prospective, multicenter US investigational device exemption trial: Clinical article. *J Neurosurg: Spine*. 2013; 19(2): 174–184. doi:10.3171/2013.4.SPINE12636.
11. Konno S, Kikuchi S. Prospective study of surgical treatment of degenerative spondylolisthesis: Comparison between decompression alone and decompression with Graf system stabilization. *Spine*. 2000; 25(12): 1533–1537.

Laminectomy Plus Fusion versus Laminectomy Alone for Lumbar Spondylolisthesis*

Ghogawala Z, Dziura J, Butler WE, et al. N Engl J Med 374(15):1424–1434, 2016

Reviewed by Jerry C. Ku and Jefferson R. Wilson

Research Question/Objective   Degenerative spondylolisthesis is a common cause of spinal stenosis, causing walking disability and leg pain in older adults. Previous studies have demonstrated the utility of surgical management in relieving these symptoms, but they have not clearly shown which surgical option is superior, although most surgeons in the United States opt for decompression with fusion in this scenario. The hypothesis of this randomized control study was that laminectomy plus fusion would result in greater physical health-related outcomes and lesser disability scores than laminectomy alone.

Study Design   A randomized control study was conducted, and patients from five centers were assessed for eligibility from March 2002 through August 2009. The primary outcome measure was the change in Short Form Survey (SF-36) physical component summary score at 2 years, with the minimal clinically important difference being 5 points; the secondary outcome measure was the Oswestry Disability Index (ODI), with the minimal clinically important difference being 10 points.

Sample Size   In total, 130 patients were identified as eligible, 40 declined to participate, and 44 declined to undergo randomization and were included in the observation group. Sixty-six patients underwent randomization, 35 were randomized into laminectomy, and 31 were randomized into laminectomy plus fusion.

Follow-Up   Initial clinical assessments were performed during routine outpatient visits at 1.5 and 3 months. Following this, the SF-36 and ODI surveys were mailed to patients to complete and return at 6 months and 1, 2, 3, and 4 years postoperatively.

---

* Ghogawala Z, Dziura J, Butler WE, et al. Laminectomy plus fusion versus laminectomy alone for lumbar spondylolisthesis. *N Engl J Med*. 2016; 374(15): 1424–1434.

Inclusion/Exclusion Criteria   Patients with grade I lumbar spondylolisthesis (degree of spondylolisthesis between 3 and 14 mm) with lumbar stenosis causing neurogenic claudication with or without lumbar radiculopathy were eligible for inclusion. Exclusion criteria included lumbar instability, defined as motion >3 mm at the listhesis level on flexion-extension radiographs or as judged by the enrolling surgeon based on history of mechanical back pain with axial loading of spine. Other exclusion criteria were history of previous lumbar spinal surgery, and American Society of Anesthesiologists (ASA) class IV or higher.

Intervention or Treatment Received   Patients in the laminectomy alone treatment arm received complete laminectomy with partial removal of the medial facet joint at the single level of spondylolisthesis. Patients in the laminectomy plus fusion treatment arm received the above treatment as well as implantation of pedicle screws, titanium alloy rods across the level of listhesis, and bone graft harvested from the iliac crest.

Results   There were no statistically significant between-group differences in baseline characteristics. At 2 years after surgery, the increase in the SF-36 physical-component summary score was significantly greater in laminectomy-plus-fusion group (15.2 points, 95% CI 10.9–19.5) than in the laminectomy-alone group (9.5 points, 95% CI 5.2–13.8). This was also true at the 3- and 4-year follow-up assessment (Table 31.1). According to a random-intercept logistic-regression model, the predicted rate of a minimal clinically important difference of 5 points at the 2-year follow-up was 91.9% (95% CI 73.1–97.9) among patients in the fusion group and 76.1% (95% CI 49.7–91.1) among patients in the decompression-alone group, but this difference was not statistically significant ($p = 0.18$). The differences in ODI score change were not significant, though they trended toward better outcomes in the laminectomy-plus-fusion group (Table 31.1).

Over the course of 4 years, the laminectomy-alone group had a 34% rate of reoperation, all for subsequent clinical instability at the index level as assessed by the primary surgeon, compared to 14% in the laminectomy-plus-fusion group, all done at an adjacent lumbar level for disc herniation or clinical instability. Surgical complications, blood loss, length of stay, and length of procedure were all significantly greater in the laminectomy-plus-fusion group than in the laminectomy-alone group.

Table 31.1 Primary and Secondary Outcome Measures

Changes in SF-36 Physical-Component Summary and ODI Scores from Baseline[a]

Outcome	Change from Baseline		Difference in Change, Fusion versus Decompression Alone (95% CI)	p-Value
	Decompression-Alone Group	Fusion Group		
SF-36 Physical-Component Summary Score				
Baseline[b]	34.7	31.5	NA	NA
1.5 months	6.3	5.1	−1.1 (−5.9 to 3.7)	0.64
3 months	7.7	12.2	4.5 (−0.7 to 9.7)	0.09
6 months	9.2	15.6	6.4 (1.1 to 11.7)	0.02
1 year	11.3	15.3	3.9 (−1.5 to 9.4)	0.16
2 years	9.5	15.2	5.7 (0.1 to 11.3)	0.046
3 years	7.9	15.3	7.4 (1.1 to 13.7)	0.02
4 years	7.4	14.1	6.7 (1.2 to 12.3)	0.02
ODI Score				
Baseline[b]	36.3	38.8	NA	NA
1.5 months	−15.3	−12.4	2.9 (−7.4 to 13.2)	0.58
3 months	−17.0	−22.2	−5.2 (−13.9 to 3.5)	0.24
6 months	−20.3	−25.9	−5.6 (−14.4 to 3.2)	0.21
1 year	−22.2	−26.1	−3.9 (−12.9 to 5.0)	0.38
2 years	−17.9	−26.3	−8.5 (−17.5 to 0.5)	0.06
3 years	−17.2	−21.8	−4.6 (−14.7 to 5.6)	0.37
4 years	−14.7	−23.7	−9.0 (−18.0 to 0.1)	0.05

Source: Ghogawala, Z. et al. *N Engl J Med.* 2016; 374(15): 1424–1434.
[a] Data are presented as least-squares mean values of changes in SF-36 physical-component summary scores and ODI scores from baseline at each follow-up point. Adjustment for multiplicity was not applied. NA denotes not applicable.
[b] The baseline scores shown are the mean values in the group.

Study Limitations As noted in the manuscript, there were some differences between the original trial registration and the final protocol, which may have some implications on internal validity. Initially, the change in SF-36 at both 1 and 2 years, as well as the ODI, were registered as the primary outcome variables. It was also specified that follow-up would continue through 5 years, and that a hospital-cost analysis would be conducted. Additionally, 14% of randomized participants were lost to follow-up at the 2-year mark, and 30% were lost at the 4-year mark. Third, the manuscript does not clearly state the indications for reoperation, and this would be an important discussion point because the reoperation rates in this dataset were higher than those found previously. Last, less-invasive decompression strategies, such as unilateral laminotomies, and other fusion strategies, including minimally invasive techniques, use of bone-graft extenders or bone morphogenetic protein, or interbody fusion techniques, have become more popular over the time course of the study. These newer surgical options raise the question of generalizability of this study.

CHAPTER 32

A Randomized, Controlled Trial of Fusion Surgery for Lumbar Spinal Stenosis*

Försth P, Ólafsson G, Carlsson T, et al. N Engl J Med 374(15):1413–1423, 2016

Reviewed by Jerry C. Ku and Jefferson R. Wilson

Research Question/Objective Lumbar spinal stenosis is the most common indication for spinal surgery, and studies have shown that surgical treatment in selected patients is more successful than conservative measures. The aim of this study was to investigate whether fusion surgery as an adjunct to decompression surgery resulted in better clinical outcomes than decompression alone in patients with lumbar spinal stenosis, with or without degenerative spondylolisthesis.

Study Design A multicenter randomized control trial was conducted. Patients with symptomatic lumbar stenosis were recruited from October 2006 through June 2012 from seven Swedish hospitals. Prior to randomization, patients were assessed for degenerative spondylolisthesis, defined as the presence of anterolisthesis of one vertebral body of ≥3 mm in relation to the vertebra below. The primary outcome measure was the Oswestry Disability Index (ODI) at 2 years postoperatively. Secondary outcome measures included the European Quality of Life–5 Dimensions (EQ-5D), Visual Analogue Scales (VAS) for leg and back pain, the Zurich Claudication Questionnaire, health economic evaluation, 6-minute walk test, and information about reoperation/complication rate.

Sample Size Three hundred fifty-eight patients were assessed for eligibility, and 247 patients underwent randomization. One hundred twenty-three patients, including 67 with degenerative spondylolisthesis, were assigned to the decompression-with-fusion group, and 124 patients, including 68 with degenerative spondylolisthesis, were assigned to the decompression-alone group.

Follow-Up Surveys were sent to participants before surgery and at 1, 2, and 5 years postoperatively.

---

* Försth P, Ólafsson G, Carlsson T, et al. A randomized, controlled trial of fusion surgery for lumbar spinal stenosis. *N Engl J Med.* 2016; 374(15): 1413–1423.

Inclusion/Exclusion Criteria   Patients between the age of 50 to 80 with a diagnosis of lumbar spinal stenosis, defined as pseudo-claudication in one or both legs and back pain (score on VAS > 30), who also had one or two adjacent stenotic segments (cross-sectional area of dural sac $\leq$75 mm^2 on MRI) between L2 and the sacrum, with duration of symptoms $\geq$6 months, were included in the study. Exclusion criteria were spondylolysis, degenerative lumbar scoliosis, history of previous surgery for lumbar spinal stenosis or instability, stenosis not caused by degenerative change, stenosis caused by herniated disc, other spinal conditions (e.g., ankylosing spondylitis, cancer, and other neurological disorders), history of vertebral compression fracture in the affected segments, or psychological disorders.

Intervention or Treatment Received   Patients in the decompression-alone group received decompression surgery, whereas patients in the decompression-with-fusion group received decompression with fusion. The method used for decompression or fusion was determined solely by the surgeon.

Results   There were no significant differences between the two groups in any of the preoperative variables. Among patients with preoperative degenerative spondylolisthesis, the mean degree of vertebral slip was 7.4 mm. Five patients were lost to follow-up. At the 2-year mark, there was no significant difference between the two treatment groups on the ODI score or the change in ODI score from baseline (Table 32.1). In addition, there was no significant interaction between the type of treatment and presence of spondylolisthesis, nor was there a difference in ODI score in a subgroup of patients with spondylolisthesis $\geq$7.4 mm. There were also no significant differences between the two groups in the secondary functional, pain, and quality-of-life measures (Table 32.1).

The decompression-with-fusion group had significantly greater operative time and amount of bleeding. The reoperation rate was 22% in the fusion group and 21% in the decompression-alone group. In terms of health economic evaluation, the mean direct costs of fusion were $6800 higher than decompression alone, mostly due to additional operating time, extended hospitalization, and cost of the implant. Indirect costs were similar in the two treatment groups.

Table 32.1 Primary and Secondary Outcome Measures

| | Outcomes in the Per-Protocol Population[a] | | | | | | | |
| | Absence of Degenerative Spondylolisthesis | | | | Presence of Degenerative Spondylolisthesis | | | |
Outcome	Fusion Group (n = 44)	Decompression-Alone Group (n = 51)	p-Value	Relative Risk (95% CI)	Fusion Group (n = 67)	Decompression-Alone Group (n = 66)	p-Value	Relative Risk (95% CI)
During the procedure								
Operating time—(min)	150 ± 47	80 ± 28	<0.01		149 ± 44	95 ± 40	<0.01	
Amount of bleeding—(ml)	648 ± 498	288 ± 319	<0.01		686 ± 434	311 ± 314	<0.01	
At 2 years								
ODI score	29 ± 20	27 ± 18	0.70		25 ± 19	21 ± 18	0.11	
EQ-5D score	0.62 ± 0.31	0.59 ± 0.35	0.85		0.63 ± 0.31	0.69 ± 0.28	0.20	
VAS score for back pain	41 ± 32	45 ± 31	0.66		36 ± 29	26 ± 25	0.15	
VAS score for leg pain	35 ± 31	34 ± 33	0.46		32 ± 30	29 ± 31	0.60	
ZCQ score								
Symptom severity	2.6 ± 1.0	2.5 ± 1.1	0.41		2.4 ± 0.9	2.4 ± 1.0	0.56	
Physical function	1.9 ± 0.7	1.8 ± 0.8	0.20		1.8 ± 0.8	1.7 ± 0.7	0.53	
Patient satisfaction	2.2 ± 0.9	2.1 ± 0.9	0.65		2.1 ± 0.9	1.9 ± 0.8	0.22	
Result of 6-minute walk test—(m)	417 ± 163	416 ± 130	0.38		382 ± 152	396 ± 144	0.60	

(Continued)

Table 32.1 (Continued) Primary and Secondary Outcome Measures

Outcome	Outcomes in the Per-Protocol Population[a]							
	Absence of Degenerative Spondylolisthesis				Presence of Degenerative Spondylolisthesis			
	Fusion Group (n = 44)	Decompression-Alone Group (n = 51)	p-Value	Relative Risk (95% CI)	Fusion Group (n = 67)	Decompression-Alone Group (n = 66)	p-Value	Relative Risk (95% CI)
Reporting satisfaction with the surgery—no. (%)[b]	23 (52)	27 (53)		0.99 (0.67–1.45)	43 (64)	45 (68)		0.94 (0.74–1.20)
Reporting decrease in back pain—no. (%)[c]	33 (75)	33 (65)		1.16 (0.89–1.51)	53 (79)	54 (82)		0.97 (0.82–1.14)
Reporting decrease in leg pain—no. (%)[d]	36 (82)	35 (69)		1.19 (0.94–1.50)	52 (78)	48 (73)		1.07 (0.88–1.30)
Reporting increase in walking distance—no. (%)[e]	40 (91)	41 (80)		1.13 (0.96–1.33)	59 (88)	57 (86)		1.02 (0.90–1.16)

Source: Försth P et al., *N. Engl. J. Med.* 2016; 374, 15: 1413–1423.

a Plus or minus value are means ± SD. The per-protocol analysis did not include the 14 patients who did not receive the assigned treatment and the 5 who were lost to follow-up. CI denotes confidence interval.

b In an assessment of overall satisfaction, patients responded to the following question: How do you feel about the results of your back surgery? The answer choices were "I'm satisfied," "I'm doubtful," and "I'm dissatisfied." The data reflect the number of patients who answered "I'm satisfied."

c In a global assessment of back pain, patients responded to following question: How is your back pain today compared with before the operation? The data reflect the number of patients who answered "completely gone," "greatly improved," or "somewhat improved."

d In a global assessment of leg pain, patients responded to following question: How is your leg or sciatic pain today compared with before the operation? The data reflect the number of patients who answered "completely gone," "greatly improved," or "somewhat improved."

e In an assessment of walking ability, patients responded to the following question: How far can you walk at a normal pace? The answer choices were "less than 100 m," "100 to 500 m," "0.5 to 1 km," and "more than 1 km." The data reflect the number of patients whose answers indicated an increase in walking distance from baseline.

ODI: Oswestry Disability Index; EQ-5D: European Quality of Life–5 Dimensions; VAS: Visual Analogue Scale; ZCQ: Zurich Claudication Questionnaire.

Study Limitations   First, the inclusion and exclusion criteria allowed into the study a wider, more heterogeneous study population, including those with lumbar stenosis with or without degenerative spondylolisthesis. Additionally, the degree of spondylolisthesis was not well characterized, other than noting that the average degree of slip was 7.4 mm in each treatment arm, and flexion-extension radiographs were not utilized to assess stability. Given these limitations, drawing conclusions from this study about specific disease populations may be difficult. Second, the type of fusion or decompression surgery was determined solely by the surgeon. Since the optimal procedure for fusion and decompression are not known and subject to change over time, the lack of standardization may confound the results. The thresholds for reoperation are unclear and also were determined solely by the surgeon.

Relevant Studies   The role of fusion in degenerative spondylolisthesis and spinal stenosis is a hotly debated and controversial topic. In 1991, Herkowitz and Kurz published a prospective study of 50 patients comparing decompressive laminectomy with decompressive laminectomy and concomitant intertransverse-process arthrodesis, and found significantly better results in the fusion group with respect to relief of back and leg pain.[1] Bridwell et al.[2] also found, in 1993, improved outcomes in their prospective study in the fusion group compared to the decompression-alone group. Since then, decompression with fusion has become the favored treatment of degenerative spondylolisthesis, especially following the Spine Patient Outcomes Research Trial (SPORT) study wherein surgical management outperformed nonsurgical management for patients with degenerative spondylolisthesis and spinal stenosis in terms of pain and functional outcomes, and where the majority of patients in the surgical arm were treated with laminectomy and fusion.[3] In the United States, routine use of fusion with decompression is performed in roughly half of all patients who undergo surgery for lumbar stenosis[4] and in greater than 95% of patients who undergo surgery for degenerative spondylolisthesis.[5]

More recently, however, the use of fusion in these conditions have come into question again, especially with the advent of less invasive decompressive techniques.[6] Clinical outcomes were found to be better with decompression and fusion than with fusion alone for degenerative spondylolisthesis in two systematic reviews, though the quality of evidence was low.[7,8] This should be weighed against the increased health care costs and increased risk of medical complications associated with fusion.[9]

Given this, two randomized control trials were published in the April 2016 issue of the *New England Journal of Medicine* to revisit the utility of adding fusion to decompressive surgery for degenerative spondylolisthesis and lumbar stenosis.[*,10]

---

* Försth P, Ólafsson G, Carlsson T, et al. A randomized, controlled trial of fusion surgery for lumbar spinal stenosis. *N Engl J Med.* 2016; 374(15): 1413–1423.

along with an editorial comment concluding that the addition of instrumented fusion for the treatment of most forms of lumbar spinal stenosis does not create added value for patients and might be regarded as an overcautious and unnecessary treatment.[11] Despite similar research methodologies, the conclusions drawn from these two studies were quite disparate. Ghogawala et al.,[10] in their study of stable grade I degenerative spondylolisthesis patients, concluded that there was a statistically and clinically significant improvement in SF-36, as well as a trend toward better outcomes in ODI, at the 2-year mark for the decompression-with-fusion group compared to the decompression-alone group. Furthermore, they argued that the higher rate of reoperation in the decompression-alone group may offset any health care costs saved from decompression alone without fusion. On the other hand, Försth et al.[*] assessed a more heterogenous population of patients with lumbar stenosis, with and without degenerative spondylolisthesis, and found no significant differences in clinical and functional outcomes, despite the increased costs associated with adjunctive fusion. Shortly following this, a Cochrane systematic review, which included the above two studies as well as 22 other randomized control trials for the treatment of lumbar spinal stenosis, concluded that decompression plus fusion has not been shown to be superior to decompression alone.[12]

Overall, these studies reinforce the concept that lumbar stenosis and degenerative spondylolisthesis represent a wide spectrum of disease affecting a heterogeneous population, wherein one surgical technique may not be beneficial for all patients. More research is required to delineate patient characteristics that may be predictive of which surgical technique (i.e., decompression alone versus decompression with fusion) would be best for each individual. For the time being, spine surgeons should continue to be cognizant of the idea that, while fusion is a more invasive operation with higher complication rates and longer recovery periods, it might be used to prevent the progression of listhesis and instability and to reduce the need to reoperate at that level.

REFERENCES

1. Herkowitz HN, Kurz LT. Degenerative lumbar spondylolisthesis with spinal stenosis: A prospective study comparing decompression with decompression and intertransverse process arthrodesis. *J Bone Joint Surg Am.* 1991; 73(6): 802–808.
2. Bridwell KH, Sedgewick TA, O'Brien MF, Lenke LG, Baldus C. The role of fusion and instrumentation in the treatment of degenerative spondylolisthesis with spinal stenosis. *J Spinal Disord.* 1993; 6(6): 461–472.
3. Weinstein JN, Lurie JD, Tosteson TD, et al. Surgical versus nonsurgical treatment for lumbar degenerative spondylolisthesis. *N Engl J Med.* 2007; 356(22): 2257–2270.
4. Bae HW, Rajaee SS, Kanim LE. Nationwide trends in the surgical management of lumbar spinal stenosis. *Spine (Phila Pa 1976).* 2013; 38(11): 916–926.

---

[*] Ibid.

5. Kepler CK, Vaccaro AR, Hilibrand AS, et al. National trends in the use of fusion techniques to treat degenerative spondylolisthesis. *Spine (Phila Pa 1976)*. 2014; 39(19): 1584–1589.
6. Joaquim AF, Milano JB, Ghizoni E, Patel AA. Is there a role for decompression alone for treating symptomatic degenerative lumbar spondylolisthesis? A systematic review. *Clin Spine Surg*. 2016; 29(5): 191–202.
7. Jacobs WC, Rubinstein SM, Willems PC, et al. The evidence on surgical interventions for low back disorders: An overview of systematic reviews. *Eur Spine J*. 2013; 22(9): 1936–1949.
8. Martin CR, Gruszczynski AT, Braunsfurth HA, Fallatah SM, O'Neil J, Wai EK. The surgical management of degenerative lumbar spondylolisthesis: A systematic review. *Spine (Phila Pa 1976)*. 2007; 32(16): 1791–1798.
9. Deyo RA, Mirza SK, Martin BI, Kreuter W, Goodman DC, Jarvik JG. Trends, major medical complications, and charges associated with surgery for lumbar spinal stenosis in older adults. *JAMA*. 2010; 303(13): 1259–1265.
10. Ghogawala Z, Dziura J, Butler WE, et al. Laminectomy plus fusion versus laminectomy alone for lumbar spondylolisthesis. *N Engl J Med*. 2016; 374(15): 1424–1434.
11. Peul WC, Moojen WA. Fusion for lumbar spinal stenosis: Safeguard or superfluous surgical implant? *N Engl J Med*. 2016; 374(15): 1478–1479.
12. Machado GC, Ferreira PH, Yoo RI, et al. Surgical options for lumbar spinal stenosis. *Cochrane Database Syst Rev*. 2016; 11: CD012421.

CHAPTER 33

Adolescent Idiopathic Scoliosis: A New Classification to Determine Extent of Spinal Arthrodesis*

Lenke LG, Betz RR, Harms J, et al. J Bone Joint Surg Am 83-A(8):1169–1181, 2001

Reviewed by Travis E. Marion and John T. Street

Research Question/Objective   An understanding of the three-dimensional nature and spectrum of spinal deformity is a prerequisite to the use of segmental spinal arthrodesis, and the determination of the number of levels to be fused in the management of adolescent idiopathic scoliosis (AIS). The previous King classification only considered the deformity in the coronal plane and recognized only five curve types. Furthermore, it lacked reliability and reproducibility with poor-to-fair validity.[1–3] The first objective of the proposed Lenke classification system was to create a comprehensive, easily understood, and practical system, with good-to-excellent interobserver and intraobserver reliability by utilizing objective radiographic criteria in order to consider the curve as a three-dimensional deformity. The second objective was to help standardize treatment.

Study Design   A radiographic study whereby four preoperative radiographs of the spine (standing long cassette coronal and lateral, in addition to right and left supine side bending views) from each patient were classified according to curve type (1 to 6) combined with a lumbar (A, B, or C) and sagittal thoracic spine modifier, as defined by the Scoliosis Research Society (SRS). These were reinterpreted the following day in a different sequence. Interobserver and intraobserver reliability was estimated by calculating the kappa coefficient values of simple and weighted components with 95% confidence intervals. A single observer subsequently and retrospectively applied the new Lenke system to consecutively operated patients in order to assess the prevalence of curve types.

Sample Size   Twenty-seven patients, each with four radiographs as described above, were reviewed by two groups of surgeons to determine

---

* Lenke LG, Betz RR, Harms J, et al. Adolescent idiopathic scoliosis: A new classification to determine extent of spinal arthrodesis. *J Bone Joint Surg Am.* Aug 2001; 83-A(8): 1169–1181.

interobserver and intraobserver reliability of the new Lenke system. Group 1 consisted of five surgeons, members of the SRS, involved in both the development of the new system, and the reliability testing of the King classification. Group 2 consisted of seven randomly selected members of the SRS, not previously involved in the creation of the new system. A single observer retrospectively assessed 315 consecutively operatively treated patients for the purpose of determining the prevalence of curve types.

Follow-Up   Not applicable.

Inclusion/Exclusion Criteria   Inclusion and exclusion criteria were not indicated.

Intervention or Treatment Received   Not applicable.

Results   A classification system based on three components—curve type, a lumbar modifier, and a sagittal thoracic modifier—was developed. In determining the curve type with the new classification, the mean interobserver reliability was 93% (range, 85%–100%) with a mean kappa value of 0.92 (range, 0.83–1.00) indicating good-to-excellent reliability among group 1. In reviewing the King classification, the same five reviewers revealed a mean interobserver reliability of 64%, with a mean kappa value of 0.49, indicating poor reliability. The intraobserver reliability of the new classification was 85% (range, 72%–100%), with a mean kappa value of 0.83 (range, 0.79–1.0), indicating good-to-excellent reliability, compared to the King classification, with respective values of 69% and 0.62.

For group 2, the kappa values for interobserver reliability with the new classification were 0.74 (range, 0.384–1.000) for curve type, 0.800 (0.738, 0.763, and 0.880) for the lumbar modifier, and 0.939 (0.901, 0.930, and 1.000) for the sagittal thoracic modifier. The respective values for intraobserver reliability were 0.893 (range, 0.75–1.00), 0.840 (range, 0.66–1.00), and 0.970 (range, 0.93–1.00). With the exception of curve type interobserver reliability, these values all represent good-to-excellent reliability.

In applying the new classification to the consecutive series of 315 patients, type one (main thoracic) was the most prevalent type, present in 126 (40%) of the 315. The prevalence of types 2, 3, and 5 were all 18%. The prevalence of curve type 4 (triple major) and 6 (thoracolumbar/lumbar-main thoracic) were both 3%. The prevalence of the lumbar spine modifier types A, B, and C was 30%, 21%, and 49%, respectively. The sagittal thoracic modifier revealed hypokyphosis in 18%, normal kyphosis in 71%, and hyperkyphosis in 11%.

Study Limitations   An increased element of complexity exists in creating the new Lenke system. Forty-two curve types can be derived when lumbar and thoracic sagittal modifiers are applied to 6 well-established curve types. Despite this, only 27 cases were assessed in determining the interobserver and intraobserver reliability. This number may have been inadequate. Group 2 demonstrated a lower interobserver reliability kappa score of 0.740 for curve type and a range of 0.384 to 1.000, and the results of this study could not be reproduced in subsequent studies, as detailed in the next section. A bias may exist, however, among group 1, as developers of the new Lenke system and critics of the King classification. Furthermore, in assessing prevalence of curve types, the patient population from a single referral center may not be representative of a typical practice.

The new Lenke system is not entirely comprehensive in utilizing objective criteria to consider AIS as a three-dimensional deformity. Rotation is of paramount importance when differentiating structural curves from nonstructural curves. This system was created, however, at a time when cross-sectional imaging was not universally available, and an attempt to create a reliable lumbar alignment modifier within the axial plane was not successful. Despite this, in 2001, Poncet et al. described three types of rotational deformity to assist in determining the structure of the scoliotic deformity and guide management.[4] Moreover, the new Lenke system did not address additional radiographic concepts such as lumbar lordosis, pelvic parameters, and their balance with one another.[5]

The new Lenke system was designed to standardize treatment. Only surgical management is discussed, and in focusing on curve type, it does not consider critical cosmetic components associated with AIS, such as shoulder asymmetry or rib prominence. There is no consideration for nonsurgical management.

Relevant Studies   The principal classification that preceded this study is the King classification.[1] It came under criticism for poor inter- and intraobserver reliability.[2-4] Furthermore, it had difficulty in assessing lumbar modifiers and did not account for sagittal thoracic deformity. The new Lenke system however, has since been independently assessed. When applied retrospectively to 51 radiographs, the new Lenke system was revealed to have less reliable interobserver and intraobserver reliability than initially reported, with mean kappa values of 0.62 and 0.73, respectively.[6] Richards et al. compared the reliability between the new Lenke system and the King Classification on non-premeasured radiographs of 50 patients.[7] The new Lenke system was once again found to be less reliable than initially reported. They also revealed that the interobserver and intraobserver reliability of the King classification to be good and fair, respectively, better than previously reported.

The treatment recommendations of the new system are to include structural major and minor curves within the instrumented fusion, and the nonstructural minor curves are to be excluded. An assessment of 7 operative AIS cases reviewed by 28 scoliosis surgeons resulted in high variability in selection of both operative approach and fusion level, illustrating the lack of standardized treatment paradigms at the time.[8] Puno et al. revealed, however, that the new Lenke system of classification can produce shorter fusions, and improved shoulder and trunk balance among different curves types compared to patients not classified according to the new classification.[9] Furthermore, despite the existence of variability in treatment approaches, Clements et al. and the Harms Study Group revealed that, since the implementation of the new Lenke system, there has been a reduction in variation of treatments among curve types after evaluation of prospectively collected data from a multicenter AIS study database. Ultimately, the new Lenke system has been demonstrated to classify curve patterns, allowing for successful selective thoracic or thoracolumbar fusions, with high rates of correction, while avoiding unnecessary fusions of nonstructural curves.[10-12]

REFERENCES

1. King HA, Moe JH, Bradford DS, Winter RB. The selection of fusion levels in thoracic idiopathic scoliosis. *J Bone Joint Surg Am.* 1983; 65: 1302–1313.
2. Cummings J, Loveless EA, Campbell J, et al. Interobserver reliability and intraobserver reproducibility of the system of King et al. for the classification of adolescent idiopathic scoliosis. *J Bone and Joint Surg Am.* 1998; 80: 1107–1111.
3. Lenke LG, Betz RR, Bridwell KH, et al. Intraobserver and interobserver reliability of the classification of thoracic adolescent idiopathic scoliosis. *J Bone Joint Surg Am.* 1998; 80A: 1097–1106.
4. Poncet P, Dansereau J, Labelle H. Geometric torsion in idiopathic scoliosis: Three-dimensional analysis and proposal for a new classification. *Spine.* 2001: 26; 2235–2243.
5. Tanguay F, Mac-Thiong JM, de Guise JA, et al. Relation between the sagittal pelvic and lumbar spine geometries following surgical correction of adolescent idiopathic scoliosis. *Eur Spine J.* 2007: 16; 531–536.
6. Ogon M, Giesinger K, Behensky H, et al. Interobserver and intraobserver reliability of Lenke's new scoliosis classification system. *Spine.* 2002; 27: 858–863.
7. Richards BS, Sucato DJ, Konigsberg DE, et al. Comparison of reliability between the Lenke and King classification systems for adolescent idiopathic scoliosis using radiographs that were not premeasured. *Spine.* 2003; 28: 1148–1157.
8. Lenke LG, Betz RR, Haher RT, et al. Multisurgeon assessment of surgical decision-making in adolescent idiopathic scoliosis. *Spine.* 2001; 26: 2347–2353.
9. Puno RM, An KC, Puno RL, et al. Treatment recommendations for idiopathic scoliosis: An assessment of the Lenke classification. *Spine.* 2003; 15: 2102–2112.
10. Clements DH, Marks M, Newton PO, et al. Did the Lenke classification change scoliosis treatment? *Spine.* 2011; 36: 1142–1145.
11. Lenke LG, Edwards CC, Bridwell KH. The Lenke classification of adolescent idiopathic scoliosis: How it organizes curve patterns as a template to perform selective fusions of the spine. *Spine.* 2003; 28: S199–S207.
12. Lehman RA, Lenke LG, Keeler KA, et al. Operative treatment of adolescent idiopathic scoliosis with posterior pedicle screw-only constructs: Minimum three-year follow-up of one hundred fourteen cases. *Spine.* 2008; 33: 1598–1604.

CHAPTER 34

Radiographic Analysis of Sagittal Plane Alignment and Balance in Standing Volunteers and Patients with Low Back Pain Matched for Age, Sex, and Size: A Prospective Controlled Clinical Study*

Jackson RP, McManus AC. Spine 19(14):1611–1618, 1994

Reviewed by Geoffrey Stricsek and James Harrop

Research Question/Objective   Jackson and McManus collected data for multiple spinal and pelvic parameters with the aim of exploring differences in spinopelvic alignment between individuals with and without mechanical low back pain. Additionally, given the growing utilization of spinal instrumentation, they believed their work could serve as a reference for future research evaluating the impact of instrumentation on spinal alignment and clinical outcome, including back pain.

Study Design   Prospective cohort study.

Sample Size   Two hundred total patients: 100 "patients" with mechanical low back pain, and 100 "volunteers" without back pain; there were 50 males and 50 females in each group.

Follow-Up   Not applicable.

Inclusion/Exclusion Criteria   Inclusion criteria for patients and volunteers were as follows: ages 20–65 without prior lumbar spine surgery and the absence of spondylolytic spondylolisthesis or clinical deformity. Volunteers had no significant back pain for the previous 6 months aside from an occasional, minor low backache. All patients had a chief complaint of low back pain for at least 6 weeks.

---

* Jackson R, McManus A. Radiographic analysis of sagittal plane alignment and balance in standing volunteers and patients with low back pain matched for age, sex, and size. *Spine*. 1994; 19(14): 1611–1618.

Intervention   No invasive intervention occurred. Standing 36-inch lateral X-rays were obtained for each participant and included the entire spine, pelvis, and acetabulae. The following measurements were collected: segmental and total lordosis from L1 to S1 utilizing the Cobb method; thoracic kyphosis from the superior endplate of T1 to inferior endplate of T12; thoracic apex; sagittal balance using a plumb line dropped from the center of C7 and the perpendicular distance, measured to the posterosuperior vertebral endplate of S1; sacral inclination (equivalent to sacral slope).

Results   Analog pain scores were significantly higher for patients versus volunteers. Segmental lumbar lordosis was significantly different between each motion segment across all participants; 66% of total lordosis occurred between L4 and S1. Mean total lordosis was significantly decreased in the symptomatic group (volunteers: −60.9° versus patients: −56.3°); there was no correlation with age or gender. Absolute values for segmental lordosis were significantly different between groups at the L3-L4 and L5-S1 level; however, patients had a significantly greater percentage of total lordosis localized to the L1-L2 level compared with volunteers. Sacral slope was significantly different between groups (50.4° for volunteers versus 47.2° for patients). Sacral inclination was found to be strongly correlated with segmental and total lordosis in both patients and volunteers; as segmental and total lumbar lordosis decreased, sacral slope decreased. The authors concluded that these findings were consistent with a compensatory mechanism as C7 sagittal plumb lines remained consistent between groups.

Thoracic kyphosis was not significantly different between groups. The thoracic apex was most commonly located at T7-T8 in volunteers and T6-T7 in patients; however, there was considerable variability in both groups.

There were significantly more smokers in the symptomatic group than the asymptomatic group.

Study Limitations   All measurements presented in the study were made once by a single individual using plain radiographs. Although it has been shown that manual measurement of spinopelvic parameters on plain radiographs can have excellent intra- and interobserver reliability,[1-3] the authors acknowledged that the absence of such internal controls in their study raises the question of data accuracy and consistency. Additionally, utilization of computerized methods for measurement of spinopelvic parameters has also increased since the time of publication and has been shown to provide significantly more reproducible and accurate results compared with manual techniques.[3-5]

Despite identifying a significant difference between the symptomatic and asymptomatic population, findings do not readily lend themselves to clinical application given their wide range and significant overlap; values for total lordosis ranged from −31° to −88° for volunteers, with a mean of −60.9° and standard deviation of 12.0°, and from −24° to −84° for patients, with a mean of −56.3° and standard deviation of 11.5°. Sparrey, in her review of lumbar lordosis and associated pathophysiology, observed this same variability and overlap in data and concluded that any attempt to define a threshold for a pathological condition based solely on absolute values of lumbar lordosis was "meaningless."[6]

Relevant Studies   Jackson and McManus and Stagnara[7] were some of the first to identify an association between pelvic parameters and spinal curvature, but it was Legaye's presentation of pelvic incidence that shifted the discourse surrounding measures of sagittal spinal morphology from "purely descriptive [to] analytic."[8] Pelvic incidence is an independent and constant anatomic value that is directly correlated with other pelvic parameters such as sacral slope and pelvic tilt, which in turn are significantly correlated with lumbar lordosis. Lower values of pelvic incidence have less sacral slope and, accordingly, less lumbar lordosis; a higher pelvic incidence implies greater lumbar lordosis.[8–10] Having modeled the relationship between pelvic and spinal parameters, Legaye created an equation to predict ideal lumbar lordosis based on the constant, pelvic incidence.[8] This filled a void in many prior studies that showed an association between low back pain and loss of lumbar lordosis but did not define a reference point from which any change in lumbar lordosis could actually be quantified.

Building on the work of Legaye, the Scoliosis Research Society (SRS)–Schwab criteria were crafted to look at how discrepancies between anticipated and observed spinopelvic parameters affected health-related quality of life (HRQOL) measures.[11] Linear regression models were built to identify radiographic thresholds for severe disability,[12] validated,[11] and then prospectively assessed by dividing patients into three groups based on whether lumbar lordosis was less than 10°, 10°–20°, or more than 20° of predicted value based on pelvic incidence and lumbar lordosis (PI-LL).[13] Patients who had PI-LL 10°–20° had significantly worse HRQOL compared to those with PI-LL less than 10°, and those with PI-LL greater more than 20° had significantly worse HRQOL compared with less than 10° and 10°–20°.[13] Thus, it is the relationship between pelvic incidence and lumbar lordosis that is important when assessing spinopelvic parameters for a possible biomechanical etiology of low back pain, rather than lumbar lordosis taken in isolation.

REFERENCES

1. Bredow J, Oppermann J, Scheyerer M, et al. Lumbar lordosis and sacral slope in lumbar spinal stenosis: Standard values and measurement accuracy. *Arch Orthop Surg.* 2015; 135(5): 607–612.
2. Polly DJ, Kilkelly F, McHale K, Asplund L, Mulligan M, Chang A. Measurement of lumbar lordosis: Evaluation of intraobserver, interobserver, and technique variability. *Spine (Phila Pa 1976).* 1996; 21(13): 1530–1536.

3. Wu W, Liang J, Du Y, et al. Reliability and reproducibility analysis of the Cobb angle and assessing sagittal plane by computer-assisted and manual measurement tools. *BMC Musculoskelet Disord*. 2014; 15(33).

4. Dimar J, Carreon L, Labelle H, Djurasovic M, Weidenbaum M. Intra- and inter-observer reliability of determining radiographic sagittal parameters of the spine and pelvis using a manual and a computer assisted methods. *Eur Spine J*. 2008; 17: 1373–1379.

5. Gupta M, Henry J, Schwab F, et al. Dedicated spine measurement software quantifies key spino-pelvic parameters more reliably than traditional picture archiving and communication systems tools. *Spine (Phila Pa 1976)*. 2016; 41(1): E22–E27.

6. Sparrey C, Bailey J, Safaee M, et al. Etiology of lumbar lordosis and its pathophysiology: A review of the evolution of lumbar lordosis, and the mechanics and biology of lumbar degeneration. *Neurosurg Focus*. 2014; 36(5): E1–E16.

7. Stagnara P, DeMauroy J, Dran G, et al. Reciprocal angulation of vertebral bodies in a sagittal plane: Approach to references for the evaluation of kyphosis and lordosis. *Spine*. 1982; 7(4): 335–342.

8. Legaye J, Duval-Beaupere G, Hecquet J, Marty C. Pelvic incidence: A fundamental pelvic parameter for three-dimensional regulation of spinal sagittal curves. *Eur Spine J*. 1998; 7: 99–103.

9. Boulay C, Tardieu C, Hecquet J, et al. Sagittal alignment of spine and pelvis regulated by pelvic incidence: Standard values and prediction of lordosis. *Eur Spine J*. 2006; 15: 415–422.

10. Roussouly P, Gollogly S, Berthonnaud E, Dimnet J. Classification of the normal variation in the sagittal alignment of the human lumbar spine and pelvis in the standing position. *Spine (Phila Pa 1976)*. 2005; 30(3): 346–353.

11. Schwab F, Ungar B, Blondel B, et al. Scoliosis Research Society–Schwab Adult Spinal Deformity Classification. *Spine (Phila Pa 1976)*. 2012; 37(12): 1077–1082.

12. Schwab F, Blondel B, Bess S, et al. Radiographical spinopelvic parameters and disability in the setting of adult spinal deformity: A prospective multicenter analysis. *Spine (Phila Pa 1976)*. 2013; 38(13): E803–E812.

13. Terran J, Schwab F, Shaffrey C, et al. The SRS-Schwab Adult Spinal Deformity Classification: Assessment and clinical correlations based on a prospective operative and nonoperative cohort. *Neurosurgery*. 2013; 73(4): 559–568.

CHAPTER 35

Classification of Spondylolysis and Spondylolisthesis*

Wiltse LL, Newman PH, Macnab I. Clin Orthop Relat Res 117:23–29, 1976

Reviewed by Jean-Marc Mac-Thiong

Research Question/Objective   Spondylolisthesis involves a heterogeneous group of patients with distinct anatomical features, pathophysiology, clinical presentation, and needs for treatment. Prior to the work by Wiltse et al.[†] there was no universally recognized classification of spondylolisthesis. The main objective of the current study was to describe a new classification of spondylolisthesis based on etiological and anatomical factors.

Study Design   A new classification of spondylolisthesis is presented based on clinical observations and case examples, as well as data from previous studies and expert opinions. It is also strongly influenced by their previous attempt at classifying spondylolisthesis using a different numbering system to describe the various types.[1]

Sample Size   Not applicable.

Follow-Up   Not applicable.

Inclusion/Exclusion Criteria   Not applicable.

Intervention or Treatment Received   Not applicable.

Results   The classification proposed by Wiltse et al.[‡] is divided into five types.

1. *Dysplastic*: Dysplastic spondylolisthesis refers to a congenital anomaly of the upper sacrum and posterior arch of L5 that disrupts the ability of the

---

* Wiltse LL, Newman PH, Macnab I. Classification of spondylolisis and spondylolisthesis. *Clin Orthop Relat Res*. 1976; 117: 23–29.
† Ibid.
‡ Ibid.

lumbosacral joint to withstand the loads originating from the upper body weight, thereby leading to the slippage of L5 with respect to S1. Secondary to this dysplasia, spondylolisthesis with a slippage of up to 25% can occur if the pars interarticularis remains unchanged. Otherwise, lysis and elongation of the pars interarticularis are classified as Subtypes A and B, respectively. The presence of spina bifida at L5 and/or S1 would tend to increase the risk of developing a high-grade spondylolisthesis.

2. *Isthmic*: Isthmic spondylolisthesis primarily occurs due to a lesion in the pars interarticularis, which can be one of three types. Subtype A (lytic) consists of a fatigue fracture causing separation or dissolution of the pars, most commonly occurring in children. Subtype B (elongation of the pars without separation) involves the same etiology as for Subtype A, but the absence of pars lysis is due to healing of the pars interarticularis in an elongated position following repeated fatigue microfractures. Subsequently, separation of the elongated pars interarticularis can even occur, in which case the patient is reclassified as Subtype A. As for Subtype C (acute pars fracture), a severe traumatic event is responsible for the spondylolysis with or without spondylolisthesis. Unlike Subtypes A and B, no hereditary component is involved in Subtype C.

3. *Degenerative*: Degenerative spondylolisthesis occurs after long-standing instability with remodeling and reorientation of the articular facets, and possibly multiple small compression fractures of the inferior facets of the cephalad vertebra. While increased stability at L5-S1 leads to hypermobility and increased stress at L4-L5 causes degeneration of facet joints, other risk factors include female sex, black origin, and sacralization of L5. It is seldom seen before age 50 and typically does not exceed 30%.

4. *Traumatic*: Traumatic spondylolisthesis results from an acute fracture of part of the bony hook (pedicles, pars, and facets) other than the pars interarticularis due to a severe trauma. It typically heals following nonsurgical treatment.

5. *Pathological*: In pathological spondylolisthesis, a local or generalized bone disease disrupts the ability of the bony hook to support the upper body weight without slipping.

Study Limitations   The proposed classification is mainly limited by the lack of scientific evidence and objective criteria to support the differentiation between Types I and II spondylolisthesis, and between the associated subtypes. While patients with Types III to V spondylolisthesis are distinctive and easy to classify, patients with Type I or II spondylolisthesis most often present concurrent dysplasia and pars anomaly, leading to the difficulty of accurately classifying patients. This limitation is associated with the strong reliance on anatomical/radiographic features to classify patients into Types I and II, and the difficulty of determining the etiology of spondylolisthesis only based on radiographic findings. There was no attempt at evaluating the reliability of the classification. Moreover, the classification does not include any measure of the severity of the spondylolisthesis, such that treatment guidelines cannot readily be inferred from the classification.

Relevant Studies   Marchetti and Bartolozzi[2] proposed a classification mainly based on the distinction between developmental and acquired spondylolisthesis. The acquired form includes spondylolisthesis secondary to trauma, surgery, pathological disease, or degenerative process. While they also rely on anatomical/radiographic features, Marchetti and Bartolozzi[2] introduced the concept of developmental spondylolisthesis that encompasses the Types I and II spondylolisthesis, previously described by Wiltse et al.,[2] in an attempt to provide some insight on the prognosis and treatment selection. The developmental aspect refers to a large spectrum of the condition with typical anatomical abnormalities of variable severity—similar to the concept of developmental dysplasia of the hip—rather than distinct conditions as in the classification of Wiltse et al.[2] Developmental spondylolisthesis is divided into two major types (high- and low-dysplastic), depending on the severity of bony dysplastic changes present on L5 and S1 vertebrae and on the potential risk of further slippage. The low-dysplastic type is associated with a relatively normal lumbosacral profile, a rectangular L5 vertebra, preservation of a flat upper endplate of S1, and no significant verticalization of the sacrum, and accordingly a low risk of progression. The high-dysplastic type is associated with significant lumbosacral kyphosis, trapezoidal L5 vertebra, hypoplastic/dysplastic transverse processes and posterior elements, and sacral doming with verticalization of the sacrum, and therefore a higher risk of progression. However, the developmental type described by Marchetti and Bartolozzi[2] still does not account for the wide heterogeneity in the clinical presentation of patients seen for spondylolisthesis, and their classification was not designed to guide surgical treatment. Unfortunately, the distinction between low- and high-dysplastic types is not based on strict criteria. In addition, exclusion of stress fractures of the pars interarticularis from the developmental group remains controversial since developmental spondylolisthesis also involves biomechanical factors and repetitive stresses that contribute to the spondylolisthesis, and they are difficult to distinguish clinically from a stress fracture per se.

Mac-Thiong and Labelle[3] later proposed a classification scheme for the most commonly seen form of lumbosacral spondylolisthesis for which no underlying cause has been identified, including Types I and II spondylolisthesis from the Wiltse et al. classification as well as developmental and stress fracture types from the Marchetti and Bartolozzi[2] classification. In line with the developmental concept raised by Marchetti and Bartolozzi,[2] they have organized their classification in an ascending order of severity to allow the development of an associated surgical treatment algorithm in which the complexity of the surgery increases as the severity of the spondylolisthesis increases.[3] Their classification was based on the determination of the grade of slip, degree of dysplasia, and sagittal spinopelvic balance, which are known to influence the treatment of spondylolisthesis. Through this classification, they were first to include strict quantitative criteria to classify patients with spondylolisthesis. They also emphasized the importance of measuring sagittal spinopelvic balance, following the observations of natural groupings of patients with distinct configuration of sagittal spinopelvic balance through statistical cluster and biomechanical analyses. They later excluded the need to assess the degree of dysplasia, considering that the original classification resulted in only moderate interobserver reliability mainly due to the difficulty in distinguishing between low and high dysplasia.[4] The refined classification excluding the degree of dysplasia is associated with substantial intra- and interobserver reliability.[5] In its latest version,[6] the classification (Figure 1) also includes the assessment of the lumbosacral kyphosis in order to account for its clinical relevance in spondylolisthesis.[7]

REFERENCES

1. Newman PH, Stone KH. The etiology of spondylolisthesis. *J Bone Joint Surg Br.* 1963; 45: 39–59.
2. Marchetti PC, Bartolozzi P. Classification of spondylolisthesis as a guideline for treatment. In: Bridwell KH, DeWald RL, Hammerberg KW, et al., eds. *The Textbook of Spinal Surgery,* 2nd ed. Philadelphia, PA: Lippincott-Raven; 1997: 1211–1254.
3. Mac-Thiong J-M, Labelle H. A proposal for a surgical classification of pediatric lumbosacral spondylolisthesis based on current literature. *Eur Spine J.* 2006; 15: 1425–1435.
4. Mac-Thiong J-M, Labelle H, Parent S, Hresko MT, Deviren V, Weidenbaum M, Members of the Spinal Deformity Study Group. Reliability and development of a new classification of lumbosacral spondylolisthesis. *Scoliosis.* 2008; 3: 19.
5. Mac-Thiong J-M, Duong L, Parent S, Hresko MT, Dimar JR, Weidenbaum M, Labelle H. Reliability of the Spinal Deformity Study Group classification of lumbosacral spondylolisthesis. *Spine.* 2012; 37: E95–E102.
6. Labelle H, Mac-Thiong J-M, Parent S. Section 11, Chapter 28: Surgery for pediatric spondylolisthesis. In: James M, Chapman M, eds. *Chapman's Comprehensive Orthopaedic Surgery,* 4th ed. JP Brothers Medical Publishers: 2018.
7. Tanguay F, Labelle H, Wang Z, Joncas J, de Guise JA, Mac-Thiong J-M. Clinical significance of lumbosacral kyphosis in adolescent spondylolisthesis. *Spine.* 2012; 37: 304–308.

CHAPTER 36

Scoliosis Research Society–Schwab Adult Spinal Deformity Classification: A Validation Study*

Schwab F, Ungar B, Blondel B, et al. Spine 37(12):1077–1082, 2012

Reviewed by Michael R. Bond and Tamir Ailon

Research Question/Objective   Adult spinal deformity (ASD) is a complex group of pathologies comprising a broad range of radiographic patterns and clinical presentations. A deformity classification system is needed to characterize the clinical and radiographic features, guide management, and establish a common lexicon for ASD research. The original Schwab classification system was developed based on curve type, lumbar lordosis, and amount of intervertebral subluxation in the coronal plane.[1] Recent studies have demonstrated that spinopelvic radiographic parameters are significantly correlated with health-related quality of life (HRQOL) scores. These parameters include pelvic incidence (PI), lumbar lordosis (LL), pelvic tilt (PT), and sagittal vertical axis (SVA). The aim of this study was to create and validate a classification system that incorporates these key radiographic parameters by updating and improving the current Schwab classification system.

Study Design   The authors revised a previously published classification system and conducted a validation study thereof. Sagittal radiographic modifiers were added to a modified version of the original Schwab classification. Modifier strata were determined through correlation analysis between sagittal parameters and HRQOL measures. Premarked cases were evaluated twice, approximately 1 week apart, to determine the curve type and value of THREE modifiers. Inter- and intrarater reliability for curve type and each modifier separately were assessed by calculating Fleiss's kappa coefficient.

Sample Size   Nine participants graded 21 premarked adult spine deformity cases twice each, approximately 1 week apart.

---

* Schwab F, Ungar B, Blondel B, et al. Scoliosis Research Society–Schwab Adult Spinal Deformity Classification A Validation study. *Spine*. 2012; 37(12): 1077–1082.

Follow-Up   Not applicable.

Results   The existing Schwab classification was updated to include both coronal curve type and three sagittal modifiers: PI minus LL, global alignment (SVA), and PT. Each sagittal modifier contains 3 strata (Figure 36.1). Measurements were derived from full-length anteroposterior and lateral standing radiographs. Curve types includes thoracic (T), lumbar (L) or double major curve (D) (thoracic and thoracolumbar/lumbar curves both >30), or normal (N) with no curve greater than 30°. These values were measured for each of the 21 cases and represented a range of what would have to be identified if the scoring system were to be used clinically. There were 3 patients with curve type T, 6 with type L, 7 with type D, and 5 with type N. PI-LL values ranged from −46° to 70° and included 4 patients with "0," 6 with "+," and 11 with "++." The PT ranged from 2° to 55° and had 4 patients with "0," 8 with "+," and 9 with "++." The SVA ranged from −63 to 243 mm; 11 patients had "0," 3 had "+" and 7 had "++."

Fleiss's kappa coefficient was used to analyze intrarater reliability for all radiographic parameters. With respect to intrarater reliability, the Fleiss's coefficient was classified as "almost perfect." Intrarater kappa averaged 0.94 (range, 0.70–1.0) for curve type, 0.88 (range, 0.66–1.0) for PI-LL modifier, 0.97 (range, 0.85–1.0) for PT, and 0.97 (range, 0.77–1.0) for SVA. In 87.8% of cases, the readers assigned the same overall classification on the second reading. For interrater reliability, the Fleiss's kappa coefficient improved from 0.70 to 0.79 between the first and second reading. For the curve type modifier, it improved from 0.80 to 0.87; for the PI-LL, from 0.75 to 0.86; for the PT modifier, from 0.97 to 0.98; and the SVA remained constant at 0.96. These results demonstrate that, overall, the intra- and interrater

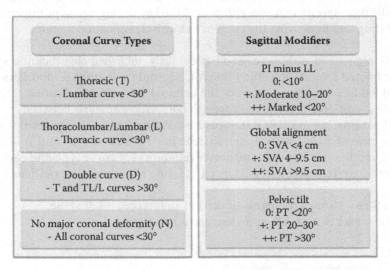

Figure 36.1   Scoliosis Research Society–Schwab Adult Spinal Deformity Classification. (From Schwab F. et al. *Spine.* 2012; 37: 1077–1082.)

reliability were excellent for the use of this classification system by members of the Scoliosis Research Society (SRS) Adult Deformity Classification committee.

Study Limitations   This study set out to evaluate the reliability of a new classification system for ASD; there were several limitations to the study that were identified. First, there were only 21 cases selected for inclusion in the study, with no mention of how they were selected or if they were representative of the range of deformity in ASD. No mention of how the cases were obtained potentially introduced selection bias. Second, the cases were "premarked," which provided evaluators with information that likely influenced the measurements they made to determine coronal curve type and sagittal modifiers. One of the challenging aspects of measuring spinopelvic parameters and coronal Cobb angles on radiographs is identifying the appropriate landmarks with precision. By providing this crucial step, the authors may have reduced variability in measurement between reviewers and thus inflated the interrater reliability. Finally, the participants were members of the SRS Adult Deformity Classification committee and were thus experts in the field. This may have further compromised the generalizability of this classification.

Relevant Studies   Classification systems for spinal deformity were originally developed for pediatric deformity. In particular, the Lenke classification[2] for adolescent idiopathic scoliosis (AIS) gained widespread acceptance. While this system was useful in the pediatric population, it does not capture the heterogeneity that is seen in ASD. Unlike children with spinal deformity, who present with concerns of curve progression and cosmesis, ASD patients typically present with pain and disability. The Schwab classification was developed to better encompass the spectrum of ASD; however, in its original conception, it did not incorporate the sagittal spino-pelvic parameters that have since come to the forefront due to their important clinical relevance.

Glassman et al. demonstrated, in a retrospective review of patients, that positive sagittal malalignment was the key radiographic driver of pain and dis-ability.[3] They also demonstrated that correction of sagittal malalignment was associated with improved clinical outcomes and that the magnitude of coronal deformity appears to be less important overall.[4] More recent studies identified that spino-pelvic parameters, including PT, SVA, PI, and LL, are more power-ful predictors of HRQOL and disability scores in patients with ASD.[5,6] This information led to the development of the SRS–Schwab classification system by including these crucial, clinically relevant parameters, and it has demonstrated overall good reliability in evaluating ASD.

One of the critiques of relying too heavily on spino-pelvic parameters is that the correlations with HRQOL that have been published are small to moderate. In an analysis of the association between positive sagittal malalignment and HRQOL, the correlation coefficients for Short Form-36, Scoliosis Research Society–22, and Oswestry Disability Index (ODI) were statistically significant but weak, ranging from 0.2 to 0.29.[3] When evaluating putative radiographic parameters for inclusion in the SRS–Schwab classification system, the highest correlation coefficients identified were for PT, SVA, and PI-LL; however, they were only 0.38, 0.47, and 0.45, respectively.[7] The specific sagittal modifier cutoffs were derived from univariate linear regression with ODI as the outcome and each sagittal modifier as the independent variable in their own separate model. The R^2 values for these models, which signify the percentage of variability in ODI accounted for by the modifier, ranged from 14% to 22%.[7] These results indicate that sagittal modifiers explain only a small portion of the variability in ODI. This suggests that there are likely a number of other factors that have an impact on HRQOL in ASD patients that are not accounted for in the SRS–Schwab classification.

Since the publication of the original article, it has been demonstrated that the SRS–Schwab classification is responsive to changes in disease severity and to surgical intervention.[8,9] More recently, a Danish group has evaluated this classification system in a prospective cohort of patients and found that the sagittal parameters were predictive of HRQOL outcomes.[10] Conversely, they demonstrated that there was no significant correlation between HRQOL and coronal curve type. In their study, the sagittal modifier cutoff points discriminated reasonably well across a variety of HRQOL measures, with the exception of PT, for which the difference between + and ++ was not significant for any HRQOL measure. The authors therefore suggest that the PT modifier cutoff points be refined. Hallager et al.[10] also demonstrated that both age and etiology of deformity (degenerative versus congenital or inflammatory) were independent predictors of HRQOL outcome. On this basis, they recommended that these factors be considered in addition to SRS–Schwab in comparative studies between different patient groups.

The study reviewed herein represents a landmark in the adult spinal deformity literature. The authors validated a classification system that is reproducible, responsive to disease severity, clinically relevant, and easy to use. The recognition of positive sagittal malalignment as the primary driver of pain and disability in ASD represents a paradigm shift in our understanding of this condition and its management. In this sense, the SRS–Schwab classification represents the culmination of several authors' work to bring sagittal radiographic parameters into the forefront of surgeons' minds when evaluating and treating ASD.

REFERENCES

1. Schwab F, Farcy JP, Bridwell K, et al. A clinical impact classification of scoliosis in the adult. *Spine*. 2006; 31: 2109–2114.
2. Lenke LG, Betz RR, Harms J, et al. Adolescent idiopathic scoliosis: A new classification to determine extent of spinal arthrodesis. *J Bone Joint Surg Am*. 2001; 83-A: 1169–1181.

3. Glassman SD, Bridwell K, Dimar J. The impact of positive sagittal balance in adult spinal deformity. *Spine*. 2005; 30(18): 2024–2029.
4. Glassman SD, Berven S, Bridwell K, et al. Correlation of radiographic parameters and clinical symptoms in adult scoliosis. *Spine*. 2005; 30(6): 682–688.
5. Lafage V, Schwab F, Patel A. Pelvic tilt and truncal inclination two key radiographic parameters in the setting of adults with spinal deformity. *Spine*. 2009; 34: E599–E606.
6. Schwab F, Lafage V, Patel A, et al. Sagittal plane considerations and the pelvis in the adult patient. *Spine*. 2009; 34(17): 1828–1833.
7. Schwab F, Blondel B, Bess S, et al. Radiographical spinopelvic parameters and disability in the setting of adult spinal deformity: A prospective multicenter analysis. *Spine*. 2013; 38(13): E803–E812.
8. Terran J, Schwab F, Shaffrey C, et al. The SRS–Schwab Adult Spinal Deformity Classification: Assessment and clinical correlations based on a prospective operative and nonoperative cohort. *Neurosurgery*. 2013; 73: 559–568.
9. Smith J, Klineberg E, Schwab F, et al. Change in classification grade by the SRS–Schwab Adult Spinal Deformity Classification predicts impact on health-related quality of life measures. *Spine*. 2013; 38(19): 1663–1671.
10. Hallager D, Hansen L, Dragsted C, et al. A comprehensive analysis of the SRS–Schwab Adult Spinal Deformity Classification and confounding variables: A prospective, non-U.S. cross-sectional study in 292 patients. *Spine*. 2015; Accepted for publication Oct 14, 2015.

CHAPTER 37

The Impact of Positive Sagittal Balance in Adult Spinal Deformity*

Glassman SD, Bridwell K, Dimar JR, et al. Spine 30:2024–2029, 2005

Reviewed by Michael M. H. Yang and W. Bradley Jacobs

Research Question/Objective Adult spinal deformity is a complex spinal disorder that, by definition, describes a spectrum of spinal disease that presents in adulthood and includes adult scoliosis, degenerative scoliosis, sagittal and coronal imbalance, and iatrogenic deformity, with or without spinal stenosis.[1] Prior to 2005, the majority of investigations of adult spinal deformity focused on the description of clinical symptoms and/or the correlation of radiographic findings with deformity or symptom progression. Unfortunately, these studies were typically limited by a lack of standardized radiographic techniques and morphometric parameters as well as a lack of validated patient-reported health status measures. This absence of clinical and radiographic standardization, combined with typically unpowered sample sizes, precluded the meaningful identification of the factors that are important to health status or treatment outcome in the adult spinal deformity population.

In an attempt to address the deficiencies of prior research studies, a multi-institutional collaboration of surgeons involved in the treatment of adult spinal deformity established a prospective database that utilized standardized radiographs and validated patient reported outcome measures. In an initial publication of this database cohort, Glassman and colleagues[2] retrospectively analyzed 298 patients with the goal of correlating radiographic measures with patient-reported outcomes. Via this analysis they were ultimately able to determine that positive sagittal balance was the radiographic parameter most highly correlated with adverse health status outcome. While this correlation had been previously identified in syndromes of postoperative sagittal imbalance, this investigation was particularly important because it was the first to identify a similar correlation in previously unoperated deformities. The sample size remained too small, however, to analyze individual factors contributing to the poor clinical tolerance to sagittal imbalance. To address this shortcoming, Glassman and

---

* Glassman SD, Bridwell K, Dimar JR, Horton W, Berven S, Schwab F. *Spine*. 2005; 30: 2024–2029.

colleagues used an expanded cohort of patients from this prospective adult spinal deformity database, with the expressed goal of identifying patients with positive sagittal balance and attempting to define the individual parameters in this population that would differentially predict clinical symptoms.

Study Design   Glassman et al. is a retrospective review of patients with adult spinal deformity enrolled in a multicenter prospective database between 2002 and 2003. Patients with positive sagittal balance were further evaluated regarding radiological parameters and health outcome measures. The health outcome measures included the Scoliosis Research Society patient questionnaire (SRS-29), MOS Short Form-12 (SF-12), and Oswestry Disability Index (ODI).

Sample Size   Of the 752 patients in the multicenter prospective database, 352 patients were identified to have a positive sagittal balance, as determined by an anterior deviation of the C7 plumb line. This positive sagittal balance group was then analyzed for parameters that may predict clinical impact.

Follow-Up   Not relevant to the Glassman et al. study because the analysis focused on the sagittal balance at enrollment and not over time or following surgical intervention.

Inclusion/Exclusion Criteria   Enrollment criteria for the prospective database were patients older than 18 years with scoliosis more than 30°, or any other significant coronal or sagittal plane spinal deformity. The cohort also included patients with spinal deformity who have undergone previous surgical correction and who were more than 18 months postoperative from the index procedure.

Intervention or Treatment Received   Not applicable because the analysis explored the effect of positive sagittal balance on patient-reported health measures at presentation and not following a specific intervention.

Results   A total of 352 patients with a positive sagittal balance were identified; 289 females and 63 males. Mean age was 54 years, and 55% of them had undergone prior spinal surgery. The two most common diagnoses were adult scoliosis in 30.4% and adult de novo scoliosis in 9.4% of cases. Kyphotic deformities, including fixed sagittal imbalance, posttraumatic kyphosis, congenital kyphosis, and Scheuermann kyphosis, comprised 20.7% of cases. The average positive sagittal balance based on C7 plumb line defined as deviation of the C7 plumb line anterior to the posterior-superior corner of S1 (Figure 37.1) ranged from 1 to 271 mm (mean 57.7 ± 51.2). The author's analysis showed a high degree of correlation between positive sagittal balance and adverse health scores for SF-12 physical health composite score (PCS) ($p < 0.000001$), SRS-29 pain domain ($p < 0.000003$), SRS-29 total ($p < 0.000001$), and ODI ($p < 0.000001$) questionnaires.

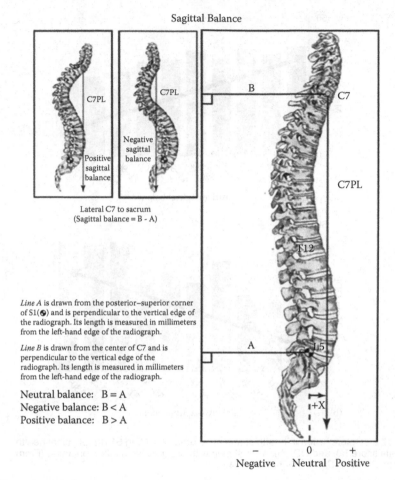

Sagittal Balance

C7PL

C7PL

Positive sagittal balance

Negative sagittal balance

B

C7

C7PL

T12

A

L5

+X

Lateral C7 to sacrum
(Sagittal balance = B - A)

Line A is drawn from the posterior–superior corner of S1(◔) and is perpendicular to the vertical edge of the radiograph. Its length is measured in millimeters from the left-hand edge of the radiograph.

Line B is drawn from the center of C7 and is perpendicular to the vertical edge of the radiograph. Its length is measured in millimeters from the left-hand edge of the radiograph.

Neutral balance: B = A
Negative balance: B < A
Positive balance: B > A

–   0   +
Negative   Neutral Positive

Figure 37.1 Technique to measure positive sagittal balance. (From Glassman SD et al. *Spine*. 2005; 30: 2024.)

Glassman et al. also showed a positive, near linear relationship between the magnitude of positive sagittal balance and increasingly adverse health outcomes. All measures of SF-12, SRS-29, and ODI showed significantly poorer scores as the C7 plumb line deviation increased (Figure 37.2). This relationship was most profound in cases with more distal (caudal) regions of maximal kyphosis. In other words, patients classified as kyphotic in the lumbar region had significantly more disability (as determined by SRS-29, and ODI, $p < 0.05$) than those with normal or lordotic lumbar sagittal Cobb measures. No correlation was found between the magnitude of positive sagittal balance and lumbar kyphosis. The authors further found no difference between thoracic or thoracolumbar sagittal Cobb deformity on any of the health status measures.

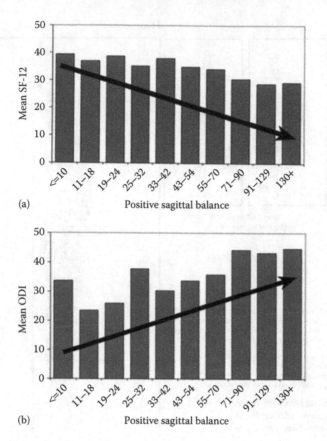

Figure 37.2 Deterioration in health status measures, including SF-12, physical health composite score (a), and ODI (b), were shown with progressive sagittal balance. (From Glassman SD et al. *Spine*. 2005; 30: 2024.)

Study Limitations   Despite the important and original findings of this manuscript, there are some noteworthy study design and implementation limitations. For instance, it is well established that there can be significant interobserver variability when measuring radiological morphometric parameters. Despite this, the authors provide no interrater reliability analysis related to the determination of the C7 plumb line. Further, the authors do not discuss the impact of technical radiographic issues such as rotation or X-ray penetration on the ability to reliably obtain required radiographic measurements. As such, the accuracy and precision of the reported radiological measurements can be questioned, thus raising some concern about the observed correlation between C7 plumb line and patient reported outcome. Second, the article does not offer health care outcome results from a control group consisting of patients with adult spinal deformity without positive sagittal balance. Without such a control group, it is difficult to ascertain the magnitude by which positive sagittal balance contributes to poorer health care outcomes. Last, the chronicity of patient symptoms and radiological deformity was not provided, which has the potential to be a significant confounder.

Relevant Studies   Historically, the majority of research studies that examined the adult spinal deformity population focused on methods to improve the radiographic appearance of deformity, with less attention paid to the effects of treatment on clinical symptoms and overall health status.[3] Studies that did attempt to correlate radiographic appearance and clinical symptoms typically suffered from a lack of standardized radiographic techniques and morphometric parameters as well as a lack of validated patient-reported health status measures.[4–7] The difficulty in determining which radiographic parameters best predicted clinical outcomes was further confounded by the lack of a rational classification system for adult spinal deformity. To address this deficiency, Schwab et al.[8] conducted a prospective study of 98 patients with adult scoliosis and ultimately identified three parameters that were consistently correlated with visual analogue pain scores: L3 end plate obliquity, frontal or coronal plane intervertebral olisthesis, and L1-S1 lordosis.[3,8] Based on these findings, the authors developed a classification system for lumbar curves based on L3 end plate obliquity and total lumbar lordosis, and their study was one of the first to show poor health outcomes correlated with specific radiological parameters.

The central importance of sagittal alignment to patient reported outcome was unequivocally defined by the two Glassman et al. manuscripts published in *Spine* in 2005.[2] As discussed previously, these studies clearly demonstrated that positive sagittal balance correlated in an essentially linear fashion with improved outcomes both in patients who had previous deformity correction surgery as well as in those that never had surgery. The authors further showed that patients with relative kyphosis in the lumbar region had significantly more disability than patients with normal or lordotic lumbar sagittal Cobb angles. Ultimately, the authors were able to conclude that maintenance or restoration of sagittal balance should be a prime goal of spinal deformity surgery.

This central importance of sagittal alignment, as purported by Glassman et al., represented a significant paradigm shift in the assessment and treatment of adult spinal deformity patients. Numerous subsequent publications have expanded on and further refined the concept of sagittal alignment in adult spinal deformity. For instance, Lafage et al.[9] further defined the importance of the pelvis, and specifically the concept of pelvis tilt, to overall sagittal alignment. Blondel et al.[10] evaluated the amount of sagittal correction needed for a patient to perceive clinically significant improvements. In this multicenter, retrospective analysis of prospectively enrolled adult spinal deformity patients, the authors showed the best health care outcomes for adult spinal deformity with severe sagittal plane deformity were obtained with a correction >120 mm of sagittal vertical axis (SVA) and at least 66% correction. Furthermore, this study showed that a larger correction corresponded to greater improvements in health care outcomes. These results are in line with the correction goals proposed by Schwab et al. for preoperative planning.[11] These studies, along with others, have ultimately lead to the recognition of the concept of spinopelvic alignment and the establishment of pelvic tilt (PT), the relationship of pelvic incidence to lumbar lordosis (PI-LL), and SVA as the major predictors of disability for adult spinal deformity patients.[12]

In conclusion, as the sophistication with which we assess and plan treatment for adult spinal deformity patients continues to evolve, it is important to recognize the seminal nature of the Glassman et al. manuscript because the restoration of appropriate sagittal alignment remains a central and fundamental tenet of the surgical treatment of patients with adult spinal deformity.

REFERENCES

1. Youssef JA, Orndorff DO, Patty CA, et al. Current status of adult spinal deformity. *Global Spine J.* 2013; 3: 51–62.
2. Glassman SD, Berven S, Bridwell K, et al. Correlation of radiographic parameters and clinical symptoms in adult scoliosis. *Spine (Phila Pa 1976).* 2005; 30: 682–688.
3. Djurasovic M, Glassman SD. Correlation of radiographic and clinical findings in spinal deformities. *Neurosurg Clin N Am.* 2007; 18: 223–227.
4. Deviren V, Berven S, Kleinstueck F, et al. Predictors of flexibility and pain patterns in thoracolumbar and lumbar idiopathic scoliosis. *Spine (Phila Pa 1976).* 2002; 27: 2346–2349.
5. Jackson RP, Simmons EH, Stripinis D. Coronal and sagittal plane spinal deformities correlating with back pain and pulmonary function in adult idiopathic scoliosis. *Spine (Phila Pa 1976).* 1989; 14: 1391–1397.
6. Schwab FJ, Smith VA, Biserni M, et al. Adult scoliosis: a quantitative radiographic and clinical analysis. *Spine (Phila Pa 1976).* 2002; 27: 387–392.
7. D'Andrea LP, Betz RR, Lenke LG, et al. Do radiographic parameters correlate with clinical outcomes in adolescent idiopathic scoliosis? *Spine (Phila Pa 1976).* 2000; 25: 1795–1802.
8. Schwab F, el-Fegoun AB, Gamez L, et al. A lumbar classification of scoliosis in the adult patient: preliminary approach. *Spine (Phila Pa 1976).* 2005; 30: 1670–1673.
9. Lafage V, Schwab F, Patel A, et al. Pelvic tilt and truncal inclination: two key radiographic parameters in the setting of adults with spinal deformity. *Spine (Phila Pa 1976).* 2009; 34: E599–E606.
10. Blondel B, Schwab F, Ungar B, et al. Impact of magnitude and percentage of global sagittal plane correction on health-related quality of life at 2-years follow-up. *Neurosurgery.* 2012; 71: 341–8; discussion 8.
11. Schwab F, Patel A, Ungar B, et al. Adult spinal deformity-postoperative standing imbalance: how much can you tolerate? An overview of key parameters in assessing alignment and planning corrective surgery. *Spine (Phila Pa 1976).* 2010; 35: 2224–2231.
12. Schwab FJ, Blondel B, Bess S, et al. Radiographical spinopelvic parameters and disability in the setting of adult spinal deformity: a prospective multicenter analysis. *Spine (Phila Pa 1976).* 2013; 38: E803–E812.
13. Glassman SD, Bridwell K, Dimar JR, et al. The impact of positive sagittal balance in adult spinal deformity. *Spine (Phila Pa 1976).* 2005; 30: 2024–2029.

The Comprehensive Anatomical Spinal Osteotomy Classification*

Schwab F. Neurosurgery 74(1):112–120, 2014

Reviewed by Ahmed Saleh and Addisu Mesfin

Research Question/Objective   Operative treatment of rigid sagittal and coronal plane deformities often requires spinal osteotomies to acquire adequate correction and provide the desired alignment. With the increase in the usage of spinal osteotomies to correct these deformities, and with no common naming or classification system in existence, a standard system was needed to classify spinal osteotomies for research purposes and to simplify communication among spinal surgeons. Prior to this study, there was no standard method of classifying osteotomies, and several names were used for the same or similar osteotomies. The central goal of the study was to devise a novel osteotomy classification system based on the anatomic features of each osteotomy.

Study Design   An osteotomy classification was proposed in this study comprised of a grading system from 1 to 6, corresponding to increasing levels of bony resection causing increased spinal destabilization. A reliability study was then performed by fellowship-trained spinal surgeons who examined clinical cases that included X-rays and operative notes. These cases were reviewed by the surgeons at two time points. The second time point was approximately 2 weeks after the first reading.

Sample Size   Eight fellowship-trained spine surgeons reviewed 16 clinical cases, including X-rays.

Follow-Up   Not applicable.

Inclusion/Exclusion Criteria   Eligibility criteria for the clinical cases included in the reliability portion of the study were not articulated within the manuscript.

Intervention   Not applicable.

---

* Schwab F, Blondel B, Chay E, et al. The comprehensive anatomical spinal osteotomy classification. *Neurosurgery.* 2014; 74(1): 112–120.

Results   A classification system based on the anatomical levels of bony resection graded 1–6 was proposed. In addition, a surgical approach modifier was also introduced in which an osteotomy is classified as performed via a posterior approach (P), or a combined anterior and posterior approach (A/P). This modifier does not signify the spinal column that was resected.

A Grade 1 osteotomy is a partial facetectomy involving the resection of the inferior facet and joint capsule at a given spinal level. This provides limited correction and requires a mobile anterior column to be effective. This osteotomy is performed via a posterior approach.

A Grade 2 osteotomy is a complete facet joint resection in which the inferior and superior facets are resected. The posterior elements, including spinous process and ligamentum flavum, may also be removed. This osteotomy also requires a mobile anterior column to be effective. A Grade 2 osteotomy is performed via a posterior approach; however, procedures that combine an anterior soft tissue release along with this osteotomy are also included.

A Grade 3 osteotomy is a resection that involves a partial wedge of the vertebral body, the pedicles, and the posterior elements. In this osteotomy, there is no resection of the disc. A Grade 3 osteotomy can be performed via a posterior approach or a combined anterior and posterior approach.

A Grade 4 osteotomy is a resection that involves a partial wedge resection of the vertebral body, posterior elements with pedicles, and at least a portion of one adjacent disc. A portion of the vertebral body remains intact in this osteotomy. A Grade 4 osteotomy can be performed via a posterior approach or a combined anterior and posterior approach.

A Grade 5 osteotomy involves the complete removal of a vertebral body and both adjacent discs. In the thoracic spine, this also includes a partial resection of the corresponding ribs. A Grade 5 osteotomy can be performed via a posterior approach or a combined anterior and posterior approach.

A Grade 6 osteotomy is any resection that extends beyond that of a Grade 5 resection but must include the resection of at least one complete vertebral body. Removal of one complete vertebral body along with a partial resection of an adjacent body or resection of several adjacent vertebral bodies is classified as a Grade 6. A Grade 6 osteotomy can be performed via a posterior approach or a combined anterior and posterior approach.

The intra- and interobserver reliability was also reported in this study. The intrarater reliability was consistent 96.8% of the time when grading the type of osteotomy, and 95.3% of the time when applying the surgical approach modifier.

The interrater reliability found that the reviewers assigned the same overall classification 87.8% of the time. This included both the grade of resection as well as the surgical modifier.

Study Limitations This study included a novel and comprehensive classification of spinal osteotomies; however, there are several limitations of the classification system that the authors address. One limitation is that it is not all-inclusive. In addition, there are some types of resection that do not neatly fit into this classification. One example of this is an osteotomy that includes removal of the posterior elements as well as a discectomy leaving the vertebral bodies intact. Another example is a partial corpectomy performed from an anterior or lateral approach where the anterior and central portion of the vertebral body, and the adjacent discs, are removed, but the lateral and posterior aspect of the body are left behind. Another limitation of the study is the limited number of reviewers and cases that were reviewed to determine the intrarater and interrater reliability. Finally, although the goal of this article was to provide a classification of the osteotomies, the authors did not attempt to provide the indications or efficacy of each of these osteotomies.

Relevant Studies There are no other studies that provide a classification system for thoracic and lumbar osteotomies. In a follow-up paper, Ames and Schwab also describe a classification system of soft tissue release and osteotomies in the cervical spine.[1] Similar to Schwab's thoracolumbar classification, this classification was graded from 1 to 7 in ascending degrees of potential spinal destabilization. The surgical approach modifier was adjusted in this classification to include approaches more common to the cervical spine. There were 6 possible surgical approach modifiers in this classification: anterior (A), posterior (P), anterior/posterior (AP), posterior/anterior (PA), anterior/posterior/anterior (APA), posterior/anterior/posterior (PAP).

A Grade 1 osteotomy included an anterior cervical discectomy and partial uncovertebral joint resection, posterior facet capsule resection, or partial facet resection.

A Grade 2 osteotomy included resection of both superior and inferior facets at a given segment. Resection of the other components of the posterior elements such as lamina and spinous processes may also be resected.

A Grade 3 osteotomy included a partial or complete corpectomy with resection of the adjacent discs.

A Grade 4 osteotomy included an anterior osteotomy through the body and the bilateral uncovertebral joints into the transverse foramen.

A Grade 5 osteotomy included resection of all the posterior elements, including the facets, lamina, and spinous processes, along with the creation of a fracture or anterior wedge in the anterior column.

A Grade 6 osteotomy included the resection of all the posterior elements, including the facets, lamina, and spinous processes, along with removal of the pedicles and the creation of a closing wedge through the vertebral body.

A Grade 7 osteotomy included the resection of one or more entire vertebral bodies, including the adjacent discs.

The intra- and interobserver reliability was also reported in this study. Eleven readers experienced in cervical deformity reviewed 25 clinical cases. In this study, the highest-grade osteotomy performed was called the "major osteotomy," and the lower-grade osteotomies performed were called "minor osteotomies." They concluded that the intrarater reliability was "almost perfect agreement" for both the major osteotomies and the surgical approach modifier, and "moderate agreement" for the minor osteotomy. The interrater reliability was also "almost perfect agreement" for both the major osteotomies and the surgical approach modifier, and in "moderate agreement" for the minor osteotomy.

REFERENCE

1. Ames CP, Smith JS, Scheer JK, et al. A standardized nomenclature for cervical spine soft-tissue release and osteotomy for deformity correction: Clinical article. *J Neurosurg Spine*. 2013; 19: 269–278.

CHAPTER 39

The Natural History of Congenital Scoliosis*

McMaster MJ, Ohtsuka K. J Bone Joint Surg Am 64(8):1128–1147, 1982

Reviewed by Daniel J. Sucato

Research Question/Objective   Scoliosis due to congenital abnormalities of the spine is relatively uncommon and comes in a variety of different forms because the abnormalities of vertebrae come in various combinations. In addition, the locations of the abnormalities in the spine as well as the various ages of presentation, with significant growth potential in younger patients, make prediction of curve progression and therefore the need for treatment important to determine. Previous studies had incompletely defined the various combinations of congenital vertebral anatomy and the risk for progression of these curves. The main purpose of this study was to outline the natural history of congenital scoliosis in a large series of patients with detailed analysis of the types of deformity and risk factors for curve progression.

Study Design   This was a retrospective review of a large series of patients from the Edinburgh Scoliosis Clinic, which is a tertiary referral center for a large population. The patients were accrued during the years of 1958 and 1981. The patients were classified according to the previous classification of Winter et al.: unilateral unsegmented bar, unilateral unsegmented bar with contralateral hemivertebrae, block vertebra, hemivertebra, wedge vertebra and then unclassified (complex anomalies consisting of a jumble of vertebral anomalies). Each patient was followed over time to determine progression of the curve, and the rate of progression was then evaluated to determine predictive factors based on the classification, the age of the patient, and the location of the vertebral anomalies.

Sample Size   There were 251 patients with 269 curves.

Follow-Up   There were 216 patients who were followed-up for an average of 5.1 years. The remaining 35 patients were treated immediately due to

---

* McMaster MJ, Ohtsuka K. The natural history of congenital scoliosis: A study of two hundred and fifty-one patients. *J Bone Joint Surg Am.* Oct 1982; 64(8): 1128–1147.

large curves with deformity at presentation. Twelve patients were already skeletally mature with relatively small curves; treatment was not necessary and there was no follow-up because there was no risk for curve progression.

Inclusion/Exclusion Criteria All patients who presented to the Edinburgh Scoliosis Clinic during the years 1958 to 1981 who had congenital scoliosis were included. The exclusion criteria were any patient who had an underlying neuromuscular or syndromic condition.

Intervention or Treatment Received Not applicable.

Results Of the 216 patients who were followed over time, there were more females than males (179 versus 72); 108 had no treatment during the study period while the remaining 108 did not require treatment. Of the original 251 patients, 95% had a single congenital curve, while the remaining had more than one. The diagnosis of congenital scoliosis was made most commonly either in the very young age group (birth to 2 years, 30.7%) or in the older age group (between 9 and 14 years, 27.1%), and curve severity did not correlate with age of presentation. Of the 251 patients, 173 (68.9%) were seen at <10 years of age, and the average curve magnitude at presentation was evenly distributed in four groups: ≤20° (22%), 21°–39° (27%), 40°–60° (24%), and >60° (27%). The curves were classified into the following five types: 102 curves (37.9%) having a unilateral unsegmented bar, 28 (10.4%) having a bar with a contralateral hemivertebra, 13 (4.8%) having a block vertebra, 88 (32.7%) having an isolated hemivertebra, and 9 (3.3%) patients having a wedge vertebra. Twenty-nine curves were unclassified because they had multiple congenital anomalies of the spine.

The risk of progression of the curves depended on the type of deformity and the site of the curve, and there was a trend toward increasing curve severity after 10 years. For example, for the Type 1 patients with a unilateral bar who were less than 10 years, the curve progression averaged 2° per year, while those older than 10 years progressed 4° per year. The most significant progression occurred for those patients who had a unilateral unsegmented bar with a contralateral hemivertebrae in which progression was 9° per year if less than 10 years. This was followed by a unilateral unsegmented bar alone, two unilateral hemiverte-brae, a single hemivertebra, and a wedge vertebra. The region of the spine where progression was seen the most was the thoracolumbar region, followed closely by the thoracic curves and then lumbar curves; the best prognosis was for curves in the upper thoracic region.

Study Limitations This is a very well done retrospective study of a large series of patients, and the data are reported with great detail. However, there are some limitations. First, this is primarily a radiographic study without the advantage of having computed tomography (CT) to fully understand the anatomy. When seeing a patient today who has congenital scoliosis, we often obtain a CT scan to fully define the anatomy, which helps in defining risk for progression and potential treatment. Second, the risk of curve progression is somewhat biased by the fact that many of the patients had treatment either immediately or with time. Of the 251 patients, 23 patients had immediate treatment because their curve was large, while 108 patients had treatment after some progression of their curve over time. Third, there is no reporting of the outcome of treatment for these groups of patients. This does not allow the reader to understand the best way to manage the patients, the risk of complications, or the overall outcome of the various treatment modalities utilized. Finally, this study does not include lateral radiographs; therefore, sagittal plane deformity is not commented on in the study. This is very important to understand when treating patients because a concomitant sagittal plane deformity often exists, which may place more risk for progression of the curve and is important when developing strategies for correction.

Relevant Studies   The most commonly recited studies on the natural history of congenital scoliosis included the study by Winter et al., who followed 234 patients who were classified into 6 different types based on vertebral and rib morphology.[1] Progression of the curves was determined and demonstrated similar results as the current article in that unsegmented bars progressed the most; however, thoracic curves were more likely to progress when compared to other curves, including thoracolumbar curves. They reported the association between lumbar curves and anomalies of the lower extremities as well as of the genitourinary tract. More recent publications substantiate the risk of curve progression for congenital scoliosis, with greater curve progression in thoracolumbar curves followed by thoracic and then cervicothoracic curves, while patients who have unsegmented bars have higher risk, and the combination abnormalities have the highest risk.[2] Winter et al. subsequently described the follow-up of their natural history study after a posterior spinal fusion with or without Harrington instrumentation with curve correction from 55° preoperatively to 44° at follow-up. The overall results were good, with a relatively low rate of complication for bending of the fusion mass (14%), pseudoarthrosis (6.9%), and paraplegia (0.7%).[3] Three-dimensional deformity classifications may be helpful to identify more specifically these deformities and will assist in determining a specific surgical treatment plan.[4] Congenital scoliosis involving the chest wall with associated thoracic insufficiency syndrome is important to recognize because this is a life-threatening spine and chest wall deformity that requires other treatment modalities.[5-7] The surgical treatment of congenital scoliosis continues to evolve, with more aggressive surgical techniques to include three-column osteotomies and resections when appropriate. These have resulted in overall good outcomes but do carry more significant neurologic risk.[8-10]

The study by McMaster et al. set the stage for understanding the deformities and the risk of progression of these deformities, which helps guide treatment for these patients.

REFERENCES

1. Winter RB. Congenital scoliosis: A study of 234 patients treated and untreated: Part 1: natural history. *JBJS*. 1968; 50(1): 1–15.
2. Marks DS, Qaimkhani SA. The natural history of congenital scoliosis and kyphosis. *Spine*. 2009; 34(17): 1751–1755.
3. Winter RB, Moe JH, Lonstein JE. Posterior spinal arthrodesis for congenital scoliosis: An analysis of the cases of two hundred and ninety patients, five to nineteen years old. *J Bone Joint Surg Am*. 1984; 66(8): 1188–1197.
4. Kawakami N, Tsuji T, Imagama S, Lenke LG, Puno RM, Kuklo TR. Classification of congenital scoliosis and kyphosis: A new approach to the three-dimensional classification for progressive vertebral anomalies requiring operative treatment. *Spine*. 2009; 34(17): 1756–1765.
5. Campbell RM Jr., Smith MD, Mayes TC, et al. The effect of opening wedge thoracostomy on thoracic insufficiency syndrome associated with fused ribs and congenital scoliosis. *J Bone Joint Surg Am*. 2004; 86-A(8): 1659–1674.
6. Campbell RM Jr., Smith MD, Mayes TC, et al. The characteristics of thoracic insufficiency syndrome associated with fused ribs and congenital scoliosis. *J Bone Joint Surg Am*. 2003; 85-A(3): 399–408.
7. Campbell RM Jr., Hell-Vocke AK. Growth of the thoracic spine in congenital scoliosis after expansion thoracoplasty. *J Bone Joint Surg Am*. 2003; 85-A(3): 409–420.
8. Suk SI, Kim JH, Kim WJ, Lee SM, Chung ER, Nah KH. Posterior vertebral column resection for severe spinal deformities. *Spine*. 2002; 27(21): 2374–2382.
9. Ruf M, Jensen R, Letko L, Harms J. Hemivertebra resection and osteotomies in congenital spine deformity. *Spine*. 2009; 34(17): 1791–1799.
10. Hedequist DJ, Hall JE, Emans JB. Hemivertebra excision in children via simultaneous anterior and posterior exposures. *J Pediatr Orthop*. 2005; 25(1): 60–63.

CHAPTER 40

Effects of Bracing in Adolescents with Idiopathic Scoliosis*

Weinstein SL, Dolan LA, Wright JB, et al. N Engl J Med 369(16):1512–1521, 2013

Reviewed by Robert J. Ames and Amer F. Samdani

Research Question/Objective The role of bracing in adolescent idiopathic scoliosis (AIS) has been poorly defined, and controversy has persisted in regard to the efficacy of bracing. This trial was designed to investigate the efficacy of bracing compared to observation alone in preventing moderate AIS curves (20°–40°) from reaching 50° or more (i.e., surgical magnitude).

Study Design Initially designed solely as a randomized trial, the Bracing in Adolescent Idiopathic Scoliosis Trial (BRAIST) was conducted in 25 institutions across the United States and Canada. However, many families ultimately refused randomization, and a preference cohort was subsequently added to the trial. These patients were allowed to choose their own treatment. Thus, the final study design included both a randomized cohort and a preference cohort with identical inclusion criteria.

Sample Size Ultimately, 242 patients (1086 screened) were included in the primary analysis. One hundred sixteen were randomized to either bracing or observation. There were 126 patients in the preference cohort, and these patients were allowed to choose either bracing or observation.

Follow-Up Enrollment began in March 2007, and the preference group was added in November 2009. Radiographic, clinical, orthotic, and self-reported data were collected at 6-month intervals. The first interim analysis, performed in September 2012, included 178 patients. The second analysis, performed in January 2013, included 230 patients. After the second interim analysis, the data and safety monitoring board recommended early termination of the trial due to the observed efficacy of bracing.

---

* Weinstein SL, Dolan LA, Wright JG, Dobbs MB. Effects of bracing in adolescents with idiopathic scoliosis. *N Engl J Med*. 2013; 369: 1512–1521.

Inclusion/Exclusion Criteria   Patients with high-risk AIS were included in the trial. "High-risk" status was determined based on age (10–15 years), Risser score (0, 1, or 2), and Cobb angle for the largest curve (20°–40°). In addition, eligible patients could not have received any form of prior treatment for AIS.

Intervention or Treatment Received   Patients in the observation group did not receive any form of treatment or therapy. Patients in the bracing group received a rigid thoracolumbosacral orthosis (TLSO) and were instructed to wear the brace for a minimum of 18 hours per day. Compliance was monitored via a temperature logger embedded in the brace. Patients who received a brace were considered "treated" regardless of the patient's level of compliance.

Results   All clinical and radiographic outcome determinations were made at a central coordinating center by two researchers, including a research coordinator and a musculoskeletal radiologist; both were blinded to the assigned treatment. The primary outcome of the study was achieved after the first of two conditions were met: either curve progression to greater than or equal to 50° (treatment failure) or skeletal maturity prior to reaching 50° (treatment success). Maturity was defined as a Risser grade of 4 for girls (75%–100% ossification of the pelvic apophysis) and grade 5 for boys (100% ossification of the apophysis and fusion to the ilium). In addition, a minimum Sanders digital hand score of 7 was required.[1] Secondary outcomes included the Pediatric Quality of Life Inventory (PedsQL),[2,3] health and functioning,[4] self-image,[5] and perception of spinal appearance.[6] In regard to secondary outcome measures, only the PedsQL score was reported in this paper.

A total of 146 patients (60%) received a brace, while 96 patients (40%) underwent observation. In the primary analysis, the rate of treatment success was 72% in the bracing group and 48% in the observation group. After adjusting for minor differences in baseline characteristics, the calculated odds ratio for a successful outcome associated with bracing was 1.93 (95%, 1.08–3.46). The intention to treat analysis revealed similar results. The authors report a 75% success rate for bracing and 42% for observation. The number needed to treat in order to prevent one case of curve progression to surgical magnitude was 3.0.

In addition, there was a significant dose-response relationship related to bracing. Patients who wore the brace for at least 12.9 hours a day achieved a success rate of 90%–93%, while patients who wore their brace for 0–6 hours per day saw no benefit (41% success rate versus 48% in the observation alone group).

Study Limitations   In this study, 64.7% of adolescents refused to participate, and 21% of adolescents and their parents rejected randomization. The final percentage of participants that could be allocated to the randomized arm was 10.6%, including 0.9% that crossed over groups. As mentioned previously, this low inclusion rate meant that the authors altered the study into a prospective controlled trial, including a randomized arm. Thus, a limitation was the lack of complete randomization. However, due to the nature of the treatment and high rate of parental and patient preference surrounding bracing, this issue was likely unavoidable. In addition, only patients with curves 25°–40° were initially planned to be included in the trial. Due to low enrollment, however, the study expanded the inclusion criteria to include patients with curves as small as 20°. The indication for bracing these smaller curves was not expounded upon in their report (i.e., curve progression or extreme skeletal immaturity). Moreover, the effect of bracing on patients in this study was not broken down by curve magnitude, which leaves many questions unanswered, particularly in regard to patients with very small curves. In addition, some patients with curves close to 50° may eventually require surgical intervention.

Relevant Studies In comparison to Weinstein and colleagues, some prior reports have shown the efficacy of bracing to be more variable, with 18%–50% of curves progressing despite bracing.[7–12] In particular, patients less than 10 years old have had poor results with bracing, likely due to their significant skeletal immaturity and substantial growth remaining.[13] Overweight body habitus has also been shown to have a negative impact on efficacy.[14] In addition, some children can have psychosocial issues surrounding brace wear, especially those who are braced for many years. Significant stress and lower self-esteem have been reported.[15–18] Misterska et al.[16] highlighted that, for some adolescent girls, the stress associated with brace wear may be higher than the stress associated with their actual spinal deformity. Of note, Weinstein and colleagues collected data and reported on quality of life via the PedsQL score, which is a generic quality-of-life instrument used in studies of acute and chronic illness. While Weinstein et al.'s results showed no significant differences between treatment and control groups at multiple time points, they have yet to report on more specific outcomes measures in regard to health and functioning, self-image, and perception of spinal appearance.

While the above-mentioned studies that question the efficacy and/or the negative impact of bracing are generally of lower quality (i.e., nonrandomized or retrospective in nature), their results are certainly worth mentioning, especially in light of the long-standing clinical equipoise that has surrounded the issue. Prior to this report, the most convincing evidence for bracing in AIS was put forward by Nachemson and Peterson[9] in a multicenter study published in JBJS in 1995. In their multicenter prospective trial, Nachemson and Peterson reported a 74% success rate associated with bracing. Many in the field largely hailed this study as solid proof of bracing's efficacy. However, this paper has multiple limitations. First, it was not designed as a randomized controlled trial. In addition, the authors defined treatment failure as a 6° increase in Cobb angle measurement, which may have minimal clinical significance. Also, there was no compliance monitoring of these patients. Compliance is known to be a major issue with brace wear, with some studies reporting compliance as low as 20%.[19–23] Last, whereas skeletal maturity in Weinstein's report was defined as a Risser of 4 for girls and 5 for boys, and a Sanders digital hand score of 7, the maturity measurements in Nachemson's report were more ill-defined.[24]

Several other reports document the efficacy of bracing. In 1986, Emans et al.[25] reported results with the Boston brace on 295 patients. Curve progression of 5° or more was noted in only 7% of the patients during treatment, and only 11% of the patients went on to surgery. A large study by Lonstein and Winter in 1994[26] showed that bracing had a significant positive effect on the natural history of AIS, with a failure rate of 43% in braced patients versus 68% in nonbraced children. Studies utilizing the Wilmington brace have displayed favorable results as well, with only 10%–28% curve progression rates.[27-29]

While there are many questions that still need to be addressed (including quality of life outcomes and psychosocial impact, and the impact of bracing on smaller and larger curves), Weinstein and colleagues have presented the most convincing evidence to date of the efficacy of bracing in patients with AIS. Because of its robust study design and clear conclusions, this paper is considered a seminal work in the field of pediatric spinal deformity.

REFERENCES

1. Sanders JO, Browne RH, McConnell SJ, Margraf SA, Cooney TE, Finegold DN. Maturity assessment and curve progression in girls with idiopathic scoliosis. *J Bone Joint Surg Am.* 2007; 89: 64–73.
2. Varni JW, Burwinkle TM, Seid M, Skarr D. The PedsQL 4.0 as a pediatric population health measure: Feasibility, reliability, and validity. *Ambul Pediatr.* 2003; 3: 329–341.
3. Varni JW, Seid M, Kurtin PS. PedsQL 4.0: Reliability and validity of the Pediatric Quality of Life Inventory version 4.0 generic core scales in health and patient populations. *Med Care.* 2001; 39: 800–812.
4. Landgraf J, Abetz L, Ware J. *The CHQ User's Manual.* Boston: The Health Institute, New England Medical Center; 1996.
5. Petersen A, Schulenberg J, Abramowitz R, Offer D, Jarcho H. A self-image questionnaire for young adolescents (SIQYA): Reliability and validity. *J Youth Adolesc.* 1984; 13: 93–111.
6. Sanders JO, Harrast JJ, Kuklo TR, et al. The Spinal Appearance Questionnaire: Results of reliability, validity, and responsiveness testing in patients with idiopathic scoliosis. *Spine (Phila Pa 1976).* 2007; 32: 2719–2722.
7. Allington NJ, Bowen JR. Adolescent idiopathic scoliosis: Treatment with the Wilmington brace. A comparison of full-time and part-time use. *J Bone Joint Surg Am.* 1996; 78: 1056–1062.
8. Karol LA. Effectiveness of bracing in male patients with idiopathic scoliosis. *Spine (Phila Pa 1976).* 2001; 26: 2001–2005.
9. Nachemson AL, Peterson LE. Effectiveness of treatment with a brace in girls who have adolescent idiopathic scoliosis: A prospective, controlled study based on data from the Brace Study of the Scoliosis Research Society. *J Bone Joint Surg Am.* 1995; 77: 815–822.

10. Rowe DE, Bernstein SM, Riddick MF, Adler F, Emans JB, Gardner-Bonneau D. A meta-analysis of the efficacy of non-operative treatments for idiopathic scoliosis. *J Bone Joint Surg Am.* 1997; 79: 664–674.

11. Noonan KJ, Weinstein SL, Jacobson WC, Dolan LA. Use of the Milwaukee brace for progressive idiopathic scoliosis. *J Bone Joint Surg Am.* 1996; 78: 557–567.

12. Peterson LE, Nachemson AL. Prediction of progression of the curve in girls who have adolescent idiopathic scoliosis of moderate severity: Logistic regression analysis based on data from the Brace Study of the Scoliosis Research Society. *J Bone Joint Surg Am.* 1995; 77: 823–827.

13. Dimeglio A, Canavese F, Charles YP. Growth and adolescent idiopathic scoliosis: When and how much? *J Pediatr Orthop.* 2011; 31: S28–S36.

14. O'Neill PJ, Karol LA, Shindle MK, et al. Decreased orthotic effectiveness in over-weight patients with adolescent idiopathic scoliosis. *J Bone Joint Surg Am.* 2005; 87: 1069–1074.

15. Misterska E, Glowacki M, Harasymczuk J. Brace and deformity-related stress level in females with adolescent idiopathic scoliosis based on the Bad Sobernheim Stress Questionnaires. *Med Sci Monit.* 2011; 17: CR83–CR90.

16. Misterska E, Glowacki M, Latuszewska J. Female patients' and parents' assessment of deformity- and brace-related stress in the conservative treatment of adolescent idiopathic scoliosis. *Spine (Phila Pa 1976).* 2012; 37: 1218–1223.

17. Clayson D, Luz-Alterman S, Cataletto MM, Levine DB. Long-term psychological sequelae of surgically versus nonsurgically treated scoliosis. *Spine (Phila Pa 1976).* 1987; 12: 983–986.

18. Cheung KM, Cheng EY, Chan SC, Yeung KW, Luk KD. Outcome assessment of bracing in adolescent idiopathic scoliosis by the use of the SRS-22 questionnaire. *Internat Orthop.* 2007; 31: 507–511.

19. Rahman T, Bowen JR, Takemitsu M, Scott C. The association between brace compliance and outcome for patients with idiopathic scoliosis. *J Pediatr Orthop.* 2005; 24: 420–422.

20. Shaughnessy WJ. Advances in scoliosis brace treatment for adolescent idiopathic scoliosis. *Orthop Clin North Am.* 2007; 38: 469–475.

21. Katz DE, Herring A, Browne RH, Kelly DM, Birch JG. Brace wear control of curve progression in adolescent idiopathic scoliosis. *J Bone Joint Surg Am.* 2010; 92: 1343–1352.

22. Sanders JO, Newton PO, Browne RH, Katz DE, Birch JG, Herring JA. Bracing for idiopathic scoliosis: How many patients require treatment to prevent one surgery? *J Bone Joint Surg Am.* 2014; 96: 649–653.

23. Takemitsu M, Bowen JR, Rahman T, Glutting JJ, Scott CB. Compliance monitoring of brace treatment for patients with idiopathic scoliosis. *Spine (Phila Pa 1976).* 2004; 29: 2070–2074.

24. Sanders JO. Bracing reduces progression of high-risk curves in idiopathic scoliosis. *J Pediatr.* 2014; 164: 673–674.

25. Emans JB, Kaelin A, Bancel P, Hall JE, Miller ME. The Boston bracing system for idiopathic scoliosis: Follow-up results in 295 patients. *Spine (Phila Pa 1976).* 1986; 11: 792–801.

26. Lonstein JE, Winter RB. The Milwaukee brace for the treatment of adolescent idiopathic scoliosis: A review of one thousand and twenty patients. *J Bone Joint Surg Am.* 1994; 76: 1207–1221.

27. Bassett GS, Bunnell WP, MacEwen GD. Treatment of idiopathic scoliosis with the Wilmington brace: Results in patients with a twenty- to thirty-nine-degree curve. *J Bone Joint Surg Am*. 1986; 68: 602–605.
28. Bunnell WP, MacEwen GD, Jayakumar S. The use of plastic jackets in the non-operative treatment of idiopathic scoliosis: Preliminary report. *J Bone Joint Surg Am*. 1980; 62: 31–38.
29. Piazza MR, Bassett GS. Curve progression after treatment with the Wilmington brace for idiopathic scoliosis. *J Pediatr Orthop*. 1990; 10: 39–43.

CHAPTER 41

Outcomes of Operative and Nonoperative Treatment for Adult Spinal Deformity: A Prospective Multicenter, Propensity-Matched Cohort Assessment with Minimum 2-Year Follow-Up*

Smith JS, Lafage V, Shaffrey CI. Neurosurgery 78(6):851–861, 2016

Reviewed by Ryan P. McLynn and Jonathan N. Grauer

Research Question/Objective The treatment of adult spinal deformity (ASD) typically begins with nonoperative modalities, with surgery considered in patients who do not experience a satisfactory response or have progression of deformity. Studies have demonstrated that operative treatment may provide significant relief in terms of pain and disability to patients with ASD.[1-5] However, complication rates from such large surgeries are high.[†2] Although prior studies have demonstrated overall advantages of surgery for this population, the authors of the study currently being reviewed note that further support for this is needed.

The purpose of the current study was to use propensity matching to compare the 2-year outcomes of patients with ASD treated operatively versus nonoperatively based on health-related quality of life (HRQOL) and correction of deformity.

Study Design A multicenter, prospective cohort study of patients receiving treatment for ASD was conducted. Patients chose either operative or nonoperative treatment, and the particular modality of treatment, through informed consent process with their surgeon.

---

* Smith JS, Lafage V, Shaffrey CI, et al. Outcomes for operative and nonoperative treatment for adult spinal deformity: A prospective multicenter, propensity-matched cohort assessment with minimum 2-year follow-up. *Neurosurg.* 2016; 78(6): 851–861.
† Ibid.

Both unmatched and propensity matched analyses of the cohort were performed. Propensity matching is a common technique used to account for differences in characteristics of the patient groups. Demographic, radiographic, and HRQOL parameters were assessed at baseline and at minimum 2-year follow-up. Complications were assessed for the surgical group.

Sample Size   A total of 689 patient met inclusion criteria for the study (286 patients in the operative group and 403 in the nonoperative group).

Follow-Up   Patients were followed for at least 2 years.
Repeat measures of HRQOL, radiographs, and data on complications in the operative group were obtained.

The minimum follow-up period was achieved by 86% (246 out of 286) of the operative cohort and 55% (223 out of 403) of the nonoperative cohort. It is noteworthy that this represents a large loss to follow-up. Further, 38 nonoperative patients were converted to operative treatment and were not included in the analysis.

Inclusion/Exclusion Criteria   To be included in the study, patients were of age $\geq$18 years and met at least one of the following criteria: scoliosis $\geq$20°, sagittal vertical axis (SVA) $\geq$5 cm, pelvic tilt $\geq$25°, or thoracic kyphosis $\geq$60°. Patients who withdrew or were lost to follow-up within the 2-year window were not included in the analysis.

Intervention or Treatment Received   Patients chose either operative or nonoperative treatment with their surgeon through an informed consent process. There was no attempt to randomize patients to either treatment group. No standardized protocols were used for operative or nonoperative treatments. Most operative patients had posterior spinal fusion (99%), 27.3% had anterior interbody fusion procedures, 7.3% had lateral interbody fusions, 15.4% had pedicle subtraction osteotomies, and 4.5% had vertebral column resections. Nonoperative modalities were selected to best suit each patient. Common modalities included physical therapy, orthotics, pharmacologic treatments, and epidural steroid injections.

Results   At baseline, operative patients were found to have significantly greater body mass index (27.1 versus 25.5), Charlson Comorbidity Index scores (1.4 versus 0.9), prevalence of depression (24.9% versus 15.7%), and history of past spine surgery (42.6% versus 18.6%). There were no significant differences in age, sex, or smoking.

Prior to treatment, Scoliosis Research Society–Schwab classifications demonstrated no difference in coronal curve types, though the global coronal curve score was significantly worse in the operative group. Patients in the operative group had significantly worse scores on pelvic tilt, SVA, and mismatch between pelvic incidence and lumbar lordosis (PI-LL). Operative patients also had significantly worse HRQOL on Oswestry Disability Index (ODI), Short Form-36 (SF-36), Scoliosis Research Society-22r (SRS-22r), and numeric rating scores for back and leg pain (all $p < 0.001$).

Among patients undergoing surgery, at least one perioperative complication (≤ 6 weeks from surgery) occurred in 53.7% of patients, while ≥ 1 delayed complication (>6 weeks) was seen in 43.5% of patients. Overall, 71.5% of operative patients experienced one or more complications in the 2-year follow-up period.

At the minimum 2-year follow-up, patients in the operative group demonstrated significant improvement in pelvic tilt, proportion with SVA >5 cm, PI-LL, maximum coronal Cobb angle, and global coronal alignment. In contrast, the nonoperative group experienced worsening of mean PI-LL and no change in other measures.

Patients in the operative group also demonstrated significant improvement in all HRQOL assessments, and the effect size was at least one minimal clinically important difference (MCID, based on values reported in previous studies) in all measures for which MCID was reported. The nonoperative group demonstrated improvements in the SRS-22r pain domain and satisfaction domain, but no change in other HRQOL measures. The proportion of patients improving by ≥ 1 MCID was significantly greater for all HRQOL measures in the operative group ($p < 0.001$).

To account for potential confounding following nonrandom assignment of patients to treatment groups, a propensity-matched analysis was performed including 97 patients from each group, matched for ODI, SRS-22r, maximum coronal Cobb angle, PI-LL, and leg pain NRS. The operative group was significantly younger (mean age, 51.4 versus 58.0 years; $p = 0.003$), but there were no significant differences in sex, body mass index (BMI), smoking, depression, Charlson Comorbidity Index (CCI), previous spine surgery, or baseline spinal deformity.

The matched operative patients had significant improvements in percentage of patients with SVA > 5 cm, PI-LL, maximum thoracolumbar/lumbar Cobb angle, and mean coronal alignment. In contrast, matched nonoperative patients demonstrated significantly worsened global coronal alignment and PI-LL, and no change in other measures.

Matched operative patients also showed significant improvement in all HRQOL measures except for SF-36 mental component, and the magnitude of all improvements was at least one MCID. Matched nonoperative patients demonstrated modest, significant improvements in SRS-22r total score and in pain and satisfaction domain scores, but no difference in other HRQOL measures.

At follow-up, the HRQOL scores were significantly superior in the operative group for all measures except SF-36 mental component.

Overall, the study demonstrates significant improvements for measures of both deformity and HRQOL in the operative group. The nonoperative group, in contrast, largely remained at baseline levels of deformity, pain, and disability. These findings were consistent in both unmatched and propensity-matched analyses. However, the operative cohort also experienced a high rate of complications.

Study Limitations   There were significant baseline differences between the operative and nonoperative groups, and patients selecting their treatments may have introduced bias in terms of patient characteristics and expectations. Propensity score matching was employed to control for differences in severity of deformity and impact of disability. While propensity matching is appropriate to minimize these confounders, it cannot fully control for individual patient decisions or other potential confounders not included in the matching. Propensity matching also created significant difference in age between the groups, which could have biased outcomes.

Additionally, follow-up rates in the nonoperative group were much lower than those in the operative group (55% as opposed to 86%). There could be significant differences between nonoperative patients who followed up and those who did not (i.e., patients with more robust improvement may have stopped seeking care), which may bias the nonoperative sample. There was no effort to compare baseline characteristics based on follow-up status.

Finally, there were no standardized protocols for operative or nonoperative treatments. Particular surgical approaches or nonsurgical modalities may have been more efficacious than others, and future studies that standardize or directly compare treatment methods would be beneficial.

Relevant Studies   The currently reviewed study's findings that operative treatment offered significant benefit to patients are consistent with other recent studies on adult spinal deformity.[1-5] In a prospective cohort study of operative versus nonoperative treatment, Bridwell and colleagues similarly found that operative patients experienced significant improvement in HRQOL scores at 2-year follow-up, while nonoperative patients did not experience significant improvement in these measures.[1] Of note, this study also experienced a poor rate of follow-up (45%) in the nonoperative group, and they observed no significant differences in gender, age, baseline back and leg pain, ODI, or SRS subscores between the follow-up and lost-to-follow-up groups. Recently, Yoshida and colleagues found that patients experienced significant improvement in SF-36, ODI, and SRS-22 at 1-year and 2-year postoperative follow-up.

It is also of note that, consistent with the currently reviewed study, high complication rates are known to occur with ASD surgery. In the currently reviewed manuscript, the authors did not investigate how complications affected HRQOL outcome measures, though prior studies have investigated this. Past studies have found that even with major complications, there tend to be significant improvements in the cohort in terms of quality-of-life measures.[2,6] Bridwell et al. found that patients with major complications experienced significant improvement in quality-of-life (QOL) measures, though it trended toward lesser improvements compared to groups with minor or no complications.[2] However, complications can increase costs and drive need for revision surgeries, and Terran and colleagues found that patients with less cost-effective treatments had poorer outcomes.[7] More research is needed to better understand the significance of this high complication rate.

REFERENCES

1. Bridwell KH, Glassman S, Horton W, et al. Does treatment (nonoperative and operative) improve the two-year quality of life in patients with adult symptomatic lumbar scoliosis? A prospective multicenter evidence-based medicine study. *Spine.* 2009; 34(20): 2171–2178.
2. Yoshida G, Boissiere L, Larrieu D, et al. Advantages and disadvantages of adult spinal deformity surgery and its impact on health-related quality of life. *Spine.* 2016. [Epub ahead of print]
3. Acaroglu E, Yavuz AC, Guler UO, et al. A decision analysis to identify the ideal treatment for adult spinal deformity: Is surgery better than non-surgical treatment in improving health-related quality of life and decreasing the disease burden? *Eur Spine J.* 2016.
4. Scheer JK, Hostin R, Robinson C, et al. Operative management of adult spinal deformity results in significant increases in QALYs gained compared to non-operative management: Analysis of 479 patients with minimum 2-year follow-up. *Spine.* 2016; [Epub ahead of print]
5. Paulus MC, Kalantar SB, Radcliff K. Cost and value of spinal deformity surgery. *Spine.* 2014; 39(5): 388–393.
6. Scheer JK, Mundis GM, Klineberg E, et al. Postoperative recovery after adult spinal deformity surgery: Comparative analysis of 149 patients during 2-year follow-up. *Spine.* 2015; 40(19): 1505–1515.
7. Terran J, McHugh BJ, Fischer CR, et al. Surgical treatment for adult spinal deformity: Projected cost effectiveness at 5-year follow-up. *Ochsner J.* 2014; 14: 14–22.

Spino-Pelvic Sagittal Balance of Spondylolisthesis: A Review and Classification*

Labelle H, Mac-Thiong Jean-Marc, Roussouly P. Eur Spine J 20:S641–S646, 2011

Reviewed by Joseph A. Osorio and Christopher P. Ames

Research Question/Objective   Spondylolisthesis occurs most commonly at the L5-S1 level, and management can involve a spectrum of interventions that include conservative treatment, instrumentation and fusion without reduction of the spondylolisthesis, and reduction with spinal realignment that includes instrumentation and fusion. There have been attempts to provide a classification scheme as a tool for the surgeon to better identify how to decide upon the various management options. Several studies have been published demonstrating the complexity of a spondylolisthesis at the L5-S1 level; several of these studies highlight that the slip alone is not the only factor that should be considered in the management of these patients.[1] Previous attempts at classifications had poor interobserver reliability; therefore, they were not adapted. The purpose of this article is to provide a classification of spondylolisthesis at the L5-S1 level that can help guide surgeons with respect to management strategy, incorporating older concepts in addition to more recent concepts surrounding spino-pelvic balance on this topic.

Study Design   A literature review article on previous L5-S1 spondylolisthesis classification systems. The review was primarily focused on work that emanated from analysis of the Spinal Deformity Study Group (SDSG) database over a 10-year period.

Sample Size   Eight hundred sixteen subjects with grade 1 to 5 spondylolisthesis from the Spinal Deformity Study Group database were included. Patient age ranged between 10 and 40 years, and the cases collected were from 43 spine surgeons in North America and Europe.

* Labelle H, Mac-Thiong JM, Roussouly P. Spino-pelvic sagittal balance of spondylolisthesis: A review and classification. *Eur Spine*. 2011; 20: S641–S646.

Follow-Up   Not applicable.

Inclusion/Exclusion Criteria   Inclusion criteria consisted of grade 1 to 5 spondylolisthesis at the L5-S1 level, for patients aged between 10 and 40 years. In addition, eligibility criteria for studies included in the review of literature were not articulated within the manuscript.

Intervention or Treatment Received   Not applicable.

Results   A classification system was defined that was based on three important characteristics determined from the lateral radiograph of the spine and pelvis: categorizing the grade of the spondylolisthesis as either low (slip <50% of vertebral body) or high (slip >50% vertebral body); measuring the pelvic incidence (PI) and classifying it as either low (less than 45°), normal (PI between 45° and 60°), or high (PI greater than 60°); and defining the pelvic balance as either balanced (high sacral slope [SS] and low pelvic tilt [PT]) or retroverted (low SS and high PT). These categories were used to define six types of L5-S1 spondylolisthesis. Type 1 was a low-grade spondylolisthesis, together with a low PI (less than 45°). Type 2 was a low-grade spondylolisthesis and normal PI (45° and 60°). Type 3 was a low-grade spondylolisthesis and PI greater than 60°. Type 4 was a high-grade spondylolisthesis, and the pelvic parameters were balanced. Type 5 was a high-grade spondylolisthesis with a retroverted pelvis that had a normal sagittal vertical axis (SVA), defined as less than 3 cm. Type 6 was a high-grade spondylolisthesis with a retroverted pelvis and a positive SVA (unbalanced spine). The progression from Type 1 to Type 6 reflects increasing associated spinal deformity, the treatment of which would ideally require restoration of the global spino-pelvic balance.

The classification system was designed to provide guidance with respect to surgical treatment. An example of this can be explained when describing a Type 4 spondylolisthesis. Patients with Type 4 spondylolisthesis display balanced alignment and a lack of spinal deformity; therefore, the author suggests that forceful attempts at reducing the deformity may not be required. In this setting, they suggest simple instrumentation and fusion after postural reduction in order to maintain the sagittal alignment. Those with a Type 5 spondylolisthesis, which they define as having a retroverted pelvis but maintaining global spinal alignment, could undergo an attempt at reduction and realignment procedures, but in difficult cases it may be sufficient to treat with simple instrumentation and fusion after postural reduction. Last, those with a Type 6 spondylolisthesis, are defined as having a spinal deformity and global spinal imbalance—here the authors felt it was mandatory that treatment should include reduction and realignment procedures to address the spinal imbalance, thus optimizing clinical outcomes and prevent treatment failure.

Study Limitations   In this study, the classification system is used to define the heterogeneity between the various types of L5-S1 spondylolisthesis as a tool toward guiding surgical treatment strategies, but the study is limited by lack of outcome data to support the proposed classification. In addition, the classification would be strengthened by showing a correlation between the severity of the spondylolisthesis and the prognosis of the patient as defined by these criteria. Second, the cohort of patients that were included for the data analysis were young in age, with patient ages ranging from 10 to 40 years of age. The age commonly encountered when treating the adult spinal deformity patient is often above this age range, and it would be important to consider this bias in the data when further describing and defining this classification system. Third, global spinal balance was defined using a sagittal vertical axis threshold measurement of 3 cm, whereas the data published on global spinal alignment defined by sagittal modifiers use 4 cm as a cutoff. Finally, although a treatment paradigm would be a valuable use from this classification system and study, this patient population is heterogeneous, and it would be best if the clinical recommendations were supported by validated outcome data.

Relevant Studies   Several studies were published prior to the discussed article provide insight for the decision-making process that preceded the classification system created by the SDSG. Hresko et al.[2] described high-grade spondylolisthesis patients as a unique entity and placed particular importance on sagittal spinal alignment that was divided into "balanced" or "unbalanced." Splitting the sagittal alignment into "balanced" and "unbalanced" was correlated with symptoms from control subjects. This study concluded that differences exist in the spondylolisthesis patient that largely have to do with whether the pelvis is balanced or unbalanced. They also suggested that reduction techniques were likely best reserved for the unbalanced subgroup.

A similar suggestion was made in the Mac-Thiong et al.[3] publication that also concluded surgical reduction for high-grade spondylolisthesis patients with postural instability as defined by lumbosacral deformity. The Labelle et al.[4] study also shared a similar argument, suggesting that high-grade spondylolisthesis patients should be subdivided into balanced and unbalanced, with the contention that reduction techniques be considered for the unbalanced retroverted pelvis subgroup.

Several years after the classification was proposed by the SDSG, Boa et al.[5] performed a validation and reliability analysis on the classification system. The results showed substantial intra- and interobserver reliability for the SDSG classification system. Their conclusion was that the classification was simple and clear, and that it provided significant clinical utility.

REFERENCES

1. Mardjetko S, Albert T, Anderson G, et al. Spine/SRS spondylolisthesis summary statement. *Spine*. 2005; 30: S3.
2. Hresko MT, Labelle H, Roussouly P, Berthonnaud E. Classification of high-grade spondylolistheses based on pelvic version and spine balance. *Spine*. 2007; 32(20): 2208–2213.
3. Mac-Thiong JM, Wang Z, de Guise JA, Labelle H. Postural model of sagittal spino-pelvic alignment and its relevance for lumbosacral developmental spondylolisthesis. *Spine*. 2008; 33(21): 2316–2325.
4. Labelle H, Roussouly P, Chopin D, Berthonnaud E, Hresko T, O'Brien M. Spino-pelvic alignment after surgical correction for developmental spondylolisthesis. *Eur Spine J*. 2008; 17: 1170–1176.
5. Boa H, Yan P, Zhu W, et al. Validation and reliability analysis of the spinal deformity study group classification for L5-S1 lumbar spondylolisthesis. *Spine*. 2015; 40(21): 1150–1154.

CHAPTER 43

The Paraspinal Sacrospinalis-Splitting Approach to the Lumbar Spine*

Wiltse LL, Bateman JG, Hutchison RF, Nelson WE.
J Bone Joint Surg Am 50(5):919–926, 1968

Reviewed by Sina Pourtaheri, Vinko Zlomislic, and Steven Garfin

Research Question/Objective   Prior to instrumented fusions, achieving fusion for L5-S1 isthmic spondylolisthesis was problematic. Wiltse et al.[†] believed that a paraspinal splitting approach would provide superior fusion rates by preserving the midline structures and allowing easy access to the posterior superior iliac spine to obtain bone graft.

Study Design   A retrospective case series of patients treated with a noninstrumented fusion via a Wiltse approach is presented in this paper. These were single-level L5-S1 fusions for isthmic spondylolisthesis. Mean age was 35 years old. The study included pediatric isthmic spondylolisthesis cases.

Sample Size   Thirty-five single-level noninstrumented lumbar fusions via a Wiltse approach.

Follow-Up   Minimum follow-up was 1 year and maximum follow-up was 7 years.

Inclusion/Exclusion Criteria   The study includes patients of all ages with a single level L5-S1 noninstrumented fusion via a Wiltse approach.

Intervention or Treatment Received   Noninstrumented fusions to the L5 transverse process and sacral ala with iliac crest bone, harvested through the same Wiltse incision. Following surgery patients were kept at bedrest in the hospital, without a brace, for 2 months postoperatively.

---

* Wiltse LL, Bateman JG, Hutchinson RH, Nelson WE. The paraspinal sacrospinalis-splitting approach to the lumbar spine. *J Bone Joint Surg Am.* 1968; 50(5): 919–926.
† Ibid.

Results   There was a 97% fusion rate (34 out of 35). The preoperative slip did not progress in the 34 patients that fused. Wiltse et al. provide illustrations for the surgical approach and bone grafting technique (see Figures 43.1 and 43.2).[*]

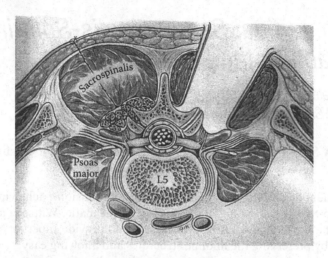

Figure 43.1   Paraspinal/sacrospinalis splitting approach. (From Wiltse, L.L. et al., *J. Bone Joint Surg. Am.*, 50, 919–926, 1968.)

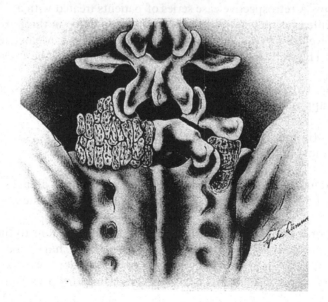

Figure 43.2   Bone-grafting technique of L5-S1 through the Wiltse approach. (From Wiltse, L.L. et al., *J. Bone Joint Surg. Am.*, 50, 919–926, 1968.)

[*] Wiltse LL, Bateman JG, Hutchinson RH, Nelson WE. The paraspinal sacrospinalis-splitting approach to the lumbar spine. *J Bone Joint Surg Am.* 1968; 50: 919–926.

Study Limitations   Retrospective case series design, without a comparison midline approach cohort.

Relevant Studies   This study was a landmark report because it provided a still-used surgical approach/technique for L5-S1 isthmic spondylolisthesis in a time of noninstrumented fusions. The primary advantage of this surgical technique in the 1960s and 1970s was preservation of midline structures to prevent further slippage and to decrease blood loss, with a high fusion rate. Wiltse et al. published, a decade later, a formal surgical technique article for this approach.[1] Wiltse et al. did not acknowledge that this approach was useful as a segmental innervation preservation of the paraspinal muscles to prevent postoperative muscle atrophy. However, several decades later the Wiltse approach has shown benefit in preventing approach-related muscle atrophy.[2] The Wiltse approach helped give birth to minimally invasive single-level and multi-level thoracolumbar fusions with or without instrumentation.[3,4]

REFERENCES

1. Wiltse LL. The paraspinal sacrospinalis-splitting approach to the lumbar spine. *Clin Orthop Relat Res.* 1973; 91: 48–57.
2. Pourtaheri S, Issa K, Lord E, et al. Paraspinal muscle atrophy after lumbar spine surgery. *Orthopedics.* 2016; 39: e209–e214.
3. Foley KT, Holly LT, Schwender JD. Minimally invasive lumbar fusion. *Spine (Phila Pa 1976).* 2003; 28: S26–S35.
4. Anand N, Baron EM, Thaiyananthan G, Khalsa K, Goldstein TB. Minimally invasive multilevel percutaneous correction and fusion for adult lumbar degenerative scoliosis: A technique and feasibility study. *J Spinal Disord Tech.* 2008; 21: 459–467.

CHAPTER 44

The Treatment of Certain Cervical-Spine Disorders by Anterior Removal of the Intervertebral Disc and Interbody Fusion*

Smith GW, Robinson RA. J Bone Joint Surg Am 40-A(3):607–624, 1958

Reviewed by Alexander Satin and Jeff Silber

Research Question/Objective   Smith and Robinson sought to accomplish three main objectives with their landmark publication. First, the authors aimed to expand on their prior work[1,2] detailing the anterior approach to the cervical spine for intervertebral disc removal and fusion. Next, the authors hoped to outline their indications for the procedure. Finally, the authors wanted to share detailed results for the first 14 patients in whom the procedure was employed. In addition to these main objectives, they shared details regarding their procedure for localization of the operative level and postoperative protocol. Prior to utilizing the procedure on humans, the authors employed eight dogs to demonstrate safety and feasibility.

Study Design   Retrospective review of patients who underwent anterior removal of cervical intervertebral discs and fusion.

Sample Size   Fourteen patients between the ages of 25 and 50 years (average 38 years). All patients were white. Five patients were men and nine were women.

Follow-Up   At the time of publication, follow-up ranged from 15 to 36 months (average 24 months).

Inclusion/Exclusion Criteria   Operative intervention was indicated in patients whose pain and disability failed to improve with conservative modalities. The authors acknowledged that posterior laminectomy is often effective in the setting of posterior osteophytes and/or acute disc protrusions. However, this technique is limited when posterior osteophytes compress nerve roots in the

---

* Smith GW, Robinson RA. The treatment of certain cervical-spine disorders by anterior removal of the intervertebral disc and interbody fusion. *J Bone Joint Surg Am.* 1958; 40-A(3): 607–624.

intervertebral foramen. To relieve nerve-root compression in the foramen, removal of the articular facet, in addition to laminectomy, may be required. This procedure, especially when employed bilaterally, can lead to cervical instability. Furthermore, removal of a degenerated but nonprolapsed cervical disc is not feasible via the posterior approach. As such, the authors state that disc removal and fusion of the cervical spine is indicated in patients whose symptoms are due to osteoarthritic spurs impinging on nerve roots in the intervertebral foramina, especially if their symptoms are bilateral or caused by disc degeneration or subluxation. Thirteen patients had clinical symptoms of cervical nerve root irritation or compression. Ten of these patients had intervertebral-disc degeneration with accompanying osteophyte formation on imaging. Three patients had disc degeneration alone without visible osteophyte formation or significant disc space narrowing. In these patients, disc degeneration was demonstrated via discography. One patient had cervical subluxation with long-tract signs due to spinal cord involvement.

Intervention or Treatment Received   Prior to the operative intervention, the authors utilized clinical and radiographic findings to identify the correct operative levels. All patients were placed in the supine position with the head turned 10° to the right. The authors preferred intranasal intubation in an effort to avoid the neck extension required to achieve mouth intubation. At the time, placing 20 pounds of cervical traction prior to incision was common practice at Johns Hopkins Hospital.

The authors utilized an 8 to 10 cm transverse incision left of the midline and about three fingerbreadths above the clavicle. The incision was carried through the skin, subcutaneous tissue, and platysma. The sternocleidomastoid muscle was retracted laterally, while the strap muscles were retracted medially and inferiorly. Next, the carotid sheath was identified with subsequent palpation of the carotid pulse. A vertical incision was then made through the paratracheal fascia medial and parallel to the carotid artery. Using their fingers, the authors spread the areolar soft tissue between the central structures (thyroid, esophagus, trachea) and the carotid sheath laterally. After careful placement of retractors, the authors identified the midline of the underlying bony structures and made a vertical incision in the prevertebral fascia.

At this point, the authors were able to identify the anterior longitudinal ligament (ALL). After placing a spinal needle in the suspected disc space, a lateral radiograph was obtained to confirm the intervertebral level. Through a small flap in the ALL, the authors removed the intervertebral-disc material and adjacent cartilage endplates using pituitary rongeurs and curettes. Large anterior osteophytes were partially removed to allow access to the disc space, but an effort was made to preserve the superior and inferior cortical bone edges, enabling the bone graft to be posteriorly countersunk. In this series, the exposed intervertebral space accepted a block of bone 10 to 15 mm high, 10 to 15 mm wide, and 10 to 15 mm deep.

To obtain the block of bone, a small incision was made over the right iliac crest. Using an osteotome, vertical cuts, 2 cm deep, roughly 2 cm apart were made at the top of the crest. The horseshoe-shaped piece of bone consisted of cancellous bone surrounded by three sides of cortical bone. The bone graft was trimmed and positioned inside the intervertebral space such that the cancellous top and bottom surfaces were in contact with the previously exposed cancellous surfaces of the endplates. After widening the intervertebral space, the bone graft was tapped into position and countersunk. After achieving hemostasis, the authors approximated the ALL. Immobilization of the neck was not utilized immediately following soft tissue closure.

In total, 22 intervertebral discs were removed and filled with bone graft. One patient had the procedure performed on three levels. Six patients had the surgery performed at two levels, and the remaining seven patients had a single-level procedure. The intervertebral disc between the fifth and sixth cervical vertebrae was most commonly removed (11), followed by the disc between the sixth and seventh cervical vertebrae (7).

Results Fusion was defined as a visible bone bridge between two vertebral bodies on imaging as well as an absence of motion between the vertebral bodies during dynamic radiographs. Of the 22 intervertebral discs operated on, 18 eventually showed a bone bridge and 21 lacked motion (three fibrous unions). Nine patients were considered to have an excellent result: all preoperative symptoms relieved. Two patients had a good result: minimal residual symptoms. Two patients had a fair result: relief of some preoperative symptoms. One patient had a poor initial result: symptoms unchanged from preoperative status.

The authors observed that neck and occipital pain was often relieved immediately after surgery. Conversely, arm pain usually disappeared after a few days.

Two patients experienced a postoperative Horner's syndrome. One case resolved after 1 week while the other resolved at 6 months. Two patients had paralysis of a vocal cord, both of which resolved. One patient had a postoperative tracheitis that resolved with conservative care. Of note, this patient had a similar complication following previous thyroid surgery, which was attributed to sensitivity to intubation tubing. The vertebral artery was perforated in one patient without sequelae. No wound infections occurred.

It is important to note that the patient who initially had a poor result was eventually reclassified as fair following an additional procedure. After fusion of the previous operative levels was noted 10 months postoperatively, she underwent multiple bilateral posterior foraminotomies and partial facetectomies, a procedure that would have resulted in instability in the absence of anterior fusion. Following the second procedure, she experienced symptom relief and was able to return to work part time.

Study Limitations The study is inherently limited by its retrospective nature and small sample size. However, given the uncertainty and technical difficulty associated with such a new procedure, the authors likely opted for a small initial patient series. Average patient follow-up was 24 months, which allowed for reasonable monitoring of postoperative pain and function. Nevertheless, this relatively short study period limited the authors' ability to report on progression of adjacent segment disease and any long-term complications.

Relevant Studies In 1955, Robinson and Smith first described the procedure for cervical intervertebral disc removal and fusion via the anterior approach.[1] This brief publication described the process by which disc degeneration and spur formation leads to cervical nerve root compression. The authors provided some conceptual support for this new procedure and early clinical data regarding eight patients. The surgical exposure was practiced on dogs prior to the first human procedure in 1954. Their surgical exposure was derived from a method used to expose esophageal diverticula.[3] In 1957, Southwick and Robinson provided a detailed anatomic approach and surgical technique for intervertebral disc removal and fusion.[2] In 1958, Cloward published a manuscript outlining a similar procedure for anterior cervical discectomy and fusion.[4] Published in the same year as the publication of interest, Cloward's paper offered similar insight into some of the limitations of the posterior cervical approach and detailed his operative technique. In the year after devising the operative technique, Cloward operated on 47 patients, achieving excellent clinical results. Of the 47 patients he operated on, 42 had complete resolution of their preoperative symptoms. In comparison to the Smith–Robinson cohort, Cloward's patients were older and predominately male. The commentary following Cloward's paper is not only entertaining but also offers some insight into how revolutionary the concept of anterior cervical fusions was at the time. In 1962, Robinson et al. published their results from 56 consecutive cases performed from 1954 to 1959, further expanding on their 1958 publication.[5] In a similar format to their previous work, the authors provided detailed illustrations of their fusion technique and shared expanded results. Their results showed that patients with more levels of degeneration had a poorer prognosis.

REFERENCES

1. Robinson RA, Smith GW. Anterolateral cervical disc removal and interbody fusion for cervical disc syndrome. *Bull Johns Hopkins Hosp.* 1955; 96: 223–224.
2. Southwick WO, Robinson RA. Surgical approaches to the vertebral bodies in the cervical and lumbar regions. *J Bone Joint Surg Am.* 1957; 39-A: 631–644.
3. Lahey FH, Warren KW. Esophageal diverticula. *Surg Gynecol Obstet.* 1954; 98: 1–28.
4. Cloward RB. The anterior approach for removal of ruptured cervical disks. *J Neurosurg.* 1958; 15: 602–617.
5. Robinson RA, Walker AE, Ferlic DC, Wiecking DK. The results of anterior interbody fusion of the cervical spine. *J Bone Joint Surg.* 1962; 44: 1569–1587.

Posterior C1-C2 Fusion with Polyaxial Screw and Rod Fixation*

Harms J, Melcher RP. Spine 26(22):2467–2471, 2001

Reviewed by David M. Brandman and Sean Barry

Research Question/Objective   Atlantoaxial instability may be caused
from a variety of etiologies, including trauma, inflammatory disorders,
and congenital malformations. Multiple techniques for fixation
had been described in the literature, consisting of either wiring and
grafting, or transarticular screw placement. The goal of this study
was to describe a novel technique for instrumentation of atlantoaxial
instability: placing C1 lateral mass and C2 pedicle polyaxial screws.

Study Design   The study describes the surgical technique in detail and
demonstrates feasibility of its use in a single-center case series.

Sample Size   Thirty-seven patients underwent instrumentation between
1997 and 2000. Mean age was 49 years (range 2–90), with 18 females.

Follow-Up   Follow-up data was available for 35 (95%) of patients, and data
was available for 27 (73%) at 6-month follow-up. No patients died in the
perioperative window.

Inclusion/Exclusion Criteria   Indications included fractures,
symptomatic os odontonium, rheumatoid arthritis, rotatory subluxations,
atlantoaxial osteoarthritis, and congenital malformations.

Intervention or Treatment Received   Patients received preoperative CT scans and
flexion-extension plain film X-rays (except in trauma patients) to demonstrate
dynamic instability at the atlantoaxial joints. Preoperative CT angiography
was performed in all patients to assess for variation in vertebral artery
location. Patients were positioned prone and held in alignment with skull

---

* Harms J, Melcher RP. Posterior C1-C2 fusion with polyaxial screw and rod fixation. *Spine.* 2001;
  26(22): 2467–2471.

tongs. Intraoperative images were taken to confirm reduction of the C1-C2 joints. Subperiosteal exposure from occiput to C3-C4 was performed, and the C1-C2 joint was exposed and used as a key reference point for C1 lateral mass screw placement. The dorsal root ganglion of C2 was exposed and retracted caudally (Figure 45.1). The authors describe cannulation of the C1 lateral masses bilaterally with a custom-made, 3.5 mm partially threaded polyaxial screw. The unthreaded portion of the screw minimizes irritation to the C2 nerve root. Polyaxial C2 pedicle screws (3.5 mm) were then placed. Intraoperative imaging was again performed to confirm correct screw placement. Further reduction of C1-C2 may be accomplished by repositioning the patient's head or manipulating the C1 or C2 screws, followed by rod fixation to maintain this improved alignment (Figure 45.2). All 37 patients underwent atlantoaxial instrumentation and fusion, and all but one were treated using soft cervical collars postoperatively.

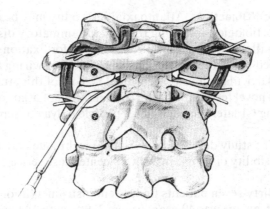

Figure 45.1   Posterior view of the upper cervical spine. The dorsal root ganglion of C2 is exposed and retracted caudally. The polyaxial screw entry points on C1 and C2 are indicated. (From Harms 2001. With permission.)

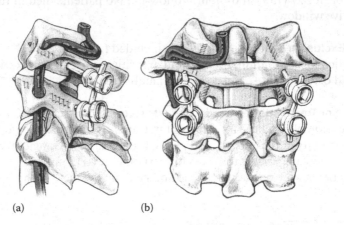

(a)   (b)

Figure 45.2   (a) Lateral, and (b) Posterior views after fixation using the polyaxial screw and rod fixation technique. (From Harms 2001. With permission.)

Results No patients had neurological deterioration or hardware failure. All patients had satisfactory screw placement and reduction. No instances of dural laceration or damage to the vertebral artery were recorded. No cases of neurologic deterioration were observed immediately postoperatively or at follow-up. Patients were followed with clinical examination and X-rays at 3 months, 6 months, and 1 year. One patient had a deep wound infection, which was treated with antibiotics and surgical debridement.

Study Limitations The case-series design, reporting positive outcomes in a small group of patients, allows the authors to comment on the feasibility of this surgical approach. Demonstration of the efficacy of this technique would require follow-up studies with larger patient numbers, longer postoperative follow-up times, and the utilization of clinically validated metrics.

Relevant Studies The approach to polyaxial screw fixation by Harms and Melcher is one of many approaches that have been described in the literature to address atlantoaxial instability.[1] Broadly speaking, fixation can be classified into either wiring and grafting, or screw fixation. Mixter and Osgood[2] were the first to describe a treatment of atlantoaxial instability by looping a silk suture between the spinous process of the axis and the posterior arch of the atlas. Gallie[3] altered this technique by placing a notched autologous bone graft between the arch of the atlas and the posterior spinous process of the axis, secured by sublaminar wires, in order to create a single midline point of fixation. However, placement of a single midline graft has the potential to act as a fulcrum between atlas and axis. Accordingly, Brooks and Jenkins[4] incorporated bilateral bone grafts affixed using 20-gauge stainless steel wires. Wire stabilization with bone grafting does not require wide lateral exposure, is not technically difficult to perform, and may be suitable for patients with unfavorable bony anatomy. However, wires must be passed through the spinal canal (which may result in iatrogenic damage to the dura or spinal cord). Moreover, patients require postoperative halo-vest immobilization to improve fusion rates;[1] early reports of this approach were associated with rates of postoperative nonunion approaching 30%.[1,5]

Screw fixation has been proposed as an alternative to wiring and grafting. Magerl and Seemann[6] first described transarticular fixation, in which a cortical screw is placed through the atlantoaxial joints bilaterally. In this study, Harms and Melcher describe their experience with polyaxial screw fixation. Since publication about it in 2001, this technique has been successfully used in thousands of patients.[5] It is worth noting that Goel and Laheri[7] described a technique for fixation of the lateral masses of the atlas and axis several years prior to that of Harms and Melcher, although their technique used stainless-steel plate and screws.

Instrumentation of the pedicle requires wide lateral exposure, of which one of the most feared complications is damage to the vertebral artery (VA). With the goal of avoiding damage to the VA, an alternative fusion technique has been described that uses C2 pars screws rather than pedicle screws. Cadaveric studies comparing these two approaches suggest greater biomechanical resistance to load failure[8] and greater insertional torque and pullout strength[9] using C2 pedicle screws versus pars screws. Recently, Elliott et al. performed a meta-analysis of 38 articles with 3380 patients[5] and found iatrogenic damage to the VA had an incidence of 0.3% and 0% for C2 pedicle and pars screws, respectively. While instrumenting the C2 pars was associated with a greater incidence of pseudarthrosis, both techniques provided excellent rates of stabilization and arthorodesis, with no statistically significant differences for radiographic or clinically significant screw malpositions.[5]

REFERENCES

1. Jacobson ME, Khan SN, An HS. C1-C2 posterior fixation: Indications, technique, and results. *Orthop Clin North Am.* 2012; 43; 11–8–vii.
2. Mixter SJ, Osgood RB IV. Traumatic lesions of the atlas and axis. *Ann Surg.* 1910; 51: 193–207.
3. Gallie WE. Fractures and dislocations of the cervical spine. *Am J Sur.* 1939; 46: 495–499.
4. Brooks AL, Jenkins EB. Atlanto-axial arthrodesis by the wedge compression method. *J Bone Joint Surg Am.* 1978; 60: 279–284.
5. Elliott RE, Tanweer O, Boah A, Smith ML, Frempong-Boadu A. Comparison of safety and stability of C-2 pars and pedicle screws for atlantoaxial fusion: Meta-analysis and review of the literature. *J Neurosurg Spine.* 2012; 17: 577–593.
6. Magerl F, Seemann PS. In *Cervical Spine I.* Springer Vienna, 1987, 322–327. doi:10.1007/978-3-7091-8882-8_59.
7. Goel A, Laheri V. Plate and screw fixation for atlanto-axial subluxation. *Acta Neurochir (Wien).* 1994; 129: 47–53.
8. Dmitriev AE, Lehman RA Jr., Helgeson MD, Sasso RC, Kuhns C, Riew DK. Acute and long-term stability of atlantoaxial fixation methods: A biomechanical comparison of pars, pedicle, and intralaminar fixation in an intact and odontoid fracture model. *Spine.* 2009; 34: 365–370.
9. Lehman RAJ, Dmitriev AE, Helgeson MD, Sasso RC, Kuklo TR, Daniel Riew K. Salvage of C2 pedicle and pars screws using the intralaminar technique: A biomechanical analysis. *Spine.* 2008; 33: 960–965.

CHAPTER 46

Pedicle Subtraction Osteotomy for the Treatment of Fixed Sagittal Imbalance*

Bridwell BH, Lewis SJ, Lenke LG, Baldus C, Blanke K.
J Bone Joint Surg Am 85-A:454–463, 2003

Reviewed by Markian A. Pahuta and Stephen J. Lewis

Research Question/Objective To analyze the clinical and radiographic outcomes for patients undergoing lumbar pedicle subtraction osteotomy (PSO).

Study Design A retrospective review of consecutive patients.

Sample Size Twenty-seven patients treated by two surgeons at one institution.

Follow-Up Two to five years.

Inclusion/Exclusion Criteria Adult patients (mean, 52.4 years; range, 32 to 70 years) treated with lumbar PSO with fixed sagittal imbalance of any etiology. The mean preoperative sagittal vertical axis (SVA) was +17.74 cm. Patients were significantly disabled by their deformity, with a mean Visual Analogue Scale (VAS) of 6.96 and an Oswestry Disability Index (ODI) score of 51.21. The etiology of sagittal imbalance included: idiopathic scoliosis ($n = 14$), degenerative deformity ($n = 8$), posttraumatic kyphosis ($n = 3$), and ankylosing spondylitis ($n = 2$). Patients had undergone a mean of 2.1 operative procedures (range, 0 to 7 procedures) prior to the index surgery.

Intervention A posterior-based lumbar PSO was performed in all patients.[1] The objective was to have the C7 plumb line fall within the L5-S1 disc or slightly behind it. The procedure was performed in two stages at the discretion of the treating surgeon.

Results The mean operative time was 12.4 hours (range, 6.8 to 18.8 hours) with mean estimated blood loss of 2396 mL (range, 500 to 6650 mL).

---

* Bridwell KH, Lewis SJ, Lenke LG, Baldus C, Blanke K. Pedicle subtraction osteotomy for the treatment of fixed sagittal imbalance. *J Bone Joint Surg Am.* 2003; 85-A: 454–463.

All patients experienced an immediate improvement in the SVA, with a mean change of −15.75 cm ($p < 0.0001$) and with a loss of 1.92 cm ($p < 0.0001$) at final follow-up. There was a mean correction of 33.52° of lordosis at the osteotomy level. There were statistically and clinically significant improvements in prospectively collected mean VAS, ODI, and Scoliosis Research Society-22 (SRS-22) scores.

One (3.7%) patient developed a pseudoarthrosis at the site of the osteotomy. One (3.7%) patient experienced a neurological injury. Three (11.1%) patients with a preoperative SVA greater than +28 cm did not have adequate correction of their sagittal imbalance through the single-level PSO.

Study Limitations   This study included patients severely disabled from a fixed deformity in their lumbar spines. The majority of these patients had noncompensated deformities with high SVAs secondary to hypolordotic lumbar spines. With these patients limited to requiring PSOs to correct their deformities, there was no control group to compare less-invasive procedures such as Smith-Petersen osteotomy, or combined anterior and posterior corrections. Furthermore, this study was published prior to our current understanding of pelvic parameters. The influence of pelvic tilt on the deformities as well as achieving a balanced relationship between the pelvic incidence and the lumbar lordosis postoperatively, which are known key determinants of clinical outcome,[2] were therefore not addressed in this series.

Relevant Studies   By reporting technical feasibility, and excellent clinical and radiographic outcomes, this article popularized the posteriorly-based PSO in the lumbar spine. Subsequent articles have reported similar results for posterior-based PSOs above and below the level of the conus.[3] PSO is now in widespread use and is a standard technique in deformity management algorithms.[4,5] Major current issues related to PSOs include indication, overcorrection, and pseudarthrosis.

In this study, Bridwell and colleagues included only patients with sagittal imbalance (deviation in SVA). However, patients with sagittal balance with sagittal malalignment (deviation in PT and/or PI-LL) may also benefit from sagittal deformity correction. *Sagittal balance* refers to whether the center of mass is centered over the pelvis and feet.[6] *Sagittal alignment* refers to whether the angular configuration of the spine permits standing with maximal muscular efficiency.[6] Even in the presence of malalignment, it is possible for the spine to be balanced due to compensatory mechanisms. Schwab and colleagues measured spinopelvic parameters in 429 adult patients with spinal deformity and determined threshold values for severe disability: PT $\geq 22°$, SVA $\geq +47$ mm, and/or PI-LL$_{T12:S1} \geq +11°$.[2] These threshold values provide a framework in planning the appropriate correction for the deformity.

The choice of osteotomy should be based on the morphology and rigidity of the deformity.[4] The magnitude of the correction should be computed from spino-pelvic parameters adjusted for age-related changes in sagittal alignment.[7,8] It is important to avoid overcorrection, which is associated with upper instrumented vertebra fractures, proximal junctional kyphosis, and negative sagittal balance. With mobile discs, multiple Smith-Petersen osteotomies (10° of lordosis per level) are preferable, allowing for similar corrections to a single PSO with less operative morbidity.[9,10]

Bone-on-bone contact of the posterior column was attempted in all cases fol-lowing osteotomy closure in this series. This contributed to a very low pseud-arthrosis rate at the level of the osteotomy of 3.7% in this study. Current studies describe techniques that involve greater posterior bone resection and leave gaps in the posterior column following osteotomy closure.[5] Use of interbody devices and multiple rods have been described as techniques to circumvent this defi-ciency. Despite these methods, pseudoarthrosis at the PSO site, which has been reported to occur in over 14% of patients,[11] continues to be a problem. Two-rod constructs and adjacent interbody fusion may lessen the rate of early rod frac-ture.[12,13] An alternative technique involves preserving the inferior facet of the cranial vertebra and the superior facet of the caudal vertebra. Reducing these structures to each other with osteotomy closure achieves direct bone apposition, restoring the integrity of the posterior column. Lewis and colleagues reported a series of 50 patients undergoing PSO with this technique and found only one pseudoarthrosis at the osteotomy site.

This study had a significant impact in demonstrating the results of pedicle subtraction osteotomies in addressing severe sagittal malalignment. With better understanding of sagittal parameters and the limitations and strengths of vari-ous osteotomies, refining of the indications and surgical techniques will further define the role of pedicle subtraction osteotomies in the treatment of fixed spinal deformities.

REFERENCES

1. Bridwell KH, et al. Pedicle subtraction osteotomy for the treatment of fixed sagittal imbalance: Surgical technique. *J Bone Joint Surg Am.* 2004; 86(Suppl A): 44–50.
2. Schwab FJ, et al. Radiographical spinopelvic parameters and disability in the setting of adult spinal deformity: A prospective multicenter analysis. *Spine (Phila Pa 1976).* 2013; 38: E803–E812.
3. O'Shaughnessy BA, et al. Thoracic pedicle subtraction osteotomy for fixed sagittal spinal deformity. *Spine (Phila Pa 1976).* 2009; 34: 2893–2899.
4. Bridwell KH. Decision making regarding Smith-Petersen vs. pedicle subtraction oste-otomy vs. vertebral column resection for spinal deformity. *Spine (Phila Pa 1976).* 2006; 31: S171–S178.

 5. Schwab F, et al. The comprehensive anatomical spinal osteotomy classification. *Neurosurgery.* 2015; 76: 112–120.
 6. Lamartina C, Berjano P. Classification of sagittal imbalance based on spinal alignment and compensatory mechanisms. *Eur Spine J.* 2014; 23: 1177–1189.
 7. Gelb DE, Lenke LG, Bridwell KH, Blanke K, McEnery KW. An analysis of sagittal spinal alignment in 100 asymptomatic middle and older aged volunteers. *Spine (Phila Pa 1976).* 1995; 20: 1351–1358.
 8. Berjano P, et al. Successful correction of sagittal imbalance can be calculated on the basis of pelvic incidence and age. *Eur Spine J.* 2014; 23(Suppl 6): 587–596.
 9. Cho KJ, Bridwell KH, Lenke LG, Berra A, Baldus C. Comparison of Smith-Petersen versus pedicle subtraction osteotomy for the correction of fixed sagittal imbalance. *Spine (Phila Pa 1976).* 2005; 30: 2030–2037; discussion 2038.
10. Lewis SJ, et al. Comparison of pedicle subtraction and Smith-Petersen osteotomies in correcting thoracic kyphosis when closed with a central hook-rod construct. *Spine (Phila Pa 1976).* 2014; 39: 1217–1224.
11. Smith JS, et al. Assessment of symptomatic rod fracture after posterior instrumented fusion for adult spinal deformity. *Neurosurgery.* 2012; 71: 862–867.
12. Gupta M, et al. Reducing rod breakage and pseudarthrosis in pedicle subtraction osteotomy: The importance of rod number and configuration in 264 patients with 2-year follow-up. *Glob Spine J.* 2016; 06.
13. Deviren V, et al. Construct rigidity after fatigue loading in pedicle subtraction osteotomy with or without adjacent interbody structural cages. *Glob Spine J.* 2012; 2: 213–220.

CHAPTER 47

Transforaminal Lumbar Interbody Fusion: Technique, Complications, and Early Results*

Rosenberg WS, Mummaneni PV. Neurosurgery 48(3):569–574, 2001

Reviewed by James Stenson and Kris Radcliff

Research Question/Objective Circumferential fusion improves rates of fusion and clinical outcomes when utilized to treat lumbosacral spine pathologies. Historically, surgeons had the choice of either a sequential two-step anterior and posterior fusion or posterior lumbar interbody fusion with simultaneous posterolateral fusion to achieve circumferential fusion. However, these approaches are fraught with their respective individual complications. The transforaminal lumbar interbody fusion (TLIF) has the potential to achieve a circumferential fusion without significant neurologic risk in a single unstaged operation. The purpose of this study was to demonstrate the safety, surgical efficacy, modifications to the technique used by the authors, and advantages of TLIF with pedicle screw fixation.

Study Design This study was a retrospective chart review of patients who underwent TLIF with combined pedicle screw fixation. The authors attempted to examine and report their findings of pain relief after surgery, intraoperative complications, infection rate, and postoperative complications. Additionally, the authors report their modifications to the previously described TLIF with segmental pedicle screw fixation.

Sample Size Twenty-two patients (12 men and 10 women) ages 34–63 years old (mean, 49 years) underwent TLIF with pedicle screw fixation. Seven of the patients were smokers. Five patients previously underwent lumbosacral spine surgery, one of which was an attempted lumbar fusion.

Follow-Up Follow-up ranged from 1 to 12 months (mean, 5.3 months).

---

* Rosenberg WS, Mummaneni PV. Transforaminal lumbar interbody fusion: Technique, complications, and early results. *Neurosurgery.* 2001; 48(3): 569–574.

Inclusion/Exclusion Criteria   The study does not specifically delineate specific inclusion criteria. However, all patients had either Grade I or II degenerative spondylolisthesis coupled with either low back pain and radiculopathy (19 patients) or low back pain only (3 patients). Exclusion criteria were not explicitly listed within the manuscript.

Intervention   Nineteen patients underwent single-level TLIF with combined pedicle screw fixation (8 patients, L4-L5; 11 patients, L5-S1). Three patients underwent two-level TLIFs with pedicle screw fixation (2 patients, L3-L4 and L4-L5; 1 patient, L4-L5 and L5-S1).

Results   Low back pain dissipated completely in 16 patients following surgery. Five patients had moderately persistent low back pain requiring oral narcotics for pain management. Last, one patient's preoperative pain level persisted postoperatively due to arachnoiditis. Fortunately, the index procedure resolved radicular symptoms in all 19 patients who presented with radiculopathy at the time of surgery. One unintentional intraoperative durotomy was noted. Primary closure was attempted at the time of durotomy, but a second more definitive operation was necessary to close the persistent CSF leak as the tear extended past the initial closure. Two postoperative wound infections were successfully treated with antibiotics and did not require revision surgery. Additional postoperative complications included transient postoperative brachial neuralgia secondary to intraoperative positioning, distal neuropathy in the arm due to prolonged blood pressure cuff inflation, and L5 motor weakness. The patient with distal arm neuropathy passed away 3 months following surgery from cardiomyopathy. The stated patient was still suffering from distal neuropathy at the time of death. The L5 motor weakness was discovered only when the patient attempted to resume jogging. Weakness resolved completely following a course of physical therapy. The authors conclude that TLIF is a safe and viable option for treatment of degenerative lumbosacral spine disease and for achieving circumferential fusion.

Study Limitations   The study is first limited due the retrospective nature of the findings. Second, the already limited sample size is further hindered by a relatively short follow-up period. Longer-term follow-up would be ideal because it takes up to 12 months for fusion rates to be determined. In addition, the pain scale was subjective. Although not intended to be an outcome study, the article would benefit from objective and validated pain and function scales such as the preoperative and postoperative Visual Analog Scale and the Oswestry Disability Index. Furthermore, patient selection was not discussed in the text, which created an inherent bias for the study pool.

Relevant Studies   TLIF with pedicle screw fixation was first described by Harms and Rolinger in 1982[1] as an alternative to the traditional two-step anterior and posterior fusion or posterior lumbar interbody fusion. TLIF allows access to the disk space via a far lateral approach after facetectomy.[2] This approach reduces the risk of neural injury, provides less dural retraction, and allows a larger interbody graft to be positioned when compared to other approaches.[3] Indications for TLIF include spondylolisthesis, symptomatic degenerative disc disease, recurrent lumbar disc herniation with significant low back pain or radiculopathy, and treatment of pseduoarthrosis.[4]

TLIF has proven to be successful in numerous studies. Chastain et al. found a statistically significant drop in both VAS (6.3 to 3.9) and Oswestry Functional Capacity (40.5%–30.0%)[5] following TLIF in patients with a minimum of 4 years follow-up. Jagannathan et al. reported evidence for correction of spondylolisthesis, restoration of sagittal balance, and improvement in disc space height when they retrospectively evaluated standing X-rays of 80 patients who underwent TLIF surgery at a minimum of 2 years follow-up.[3] In a retrospective review of 24 patients over a 3-year period, Salehi et al. demonstrated TLIF to be a safe and effective procedure when evaluating postoperative patients in terms of fusion (22 of 24 patients), Prolo score, and patient satisfaction.[6] Considered a generally safe procedure, various complications can arise before, during, and after a TLIF, including dural tear, transient radiculopathy,[7] surgical site infection,[8] hardware loosening, and persisting postoperative pain.[5]

Although the aforementioned articles report good clinical outcomes, more recent literature questions the clinical relevance of TLIF versus posterolateral fusion (PLF). Several articles have shown that functional levels and clinical outcomes do not change for patients with degenerative lumbar disorders whether an interbody fusion or posterolateral fusion is utilized.[9–11] Furthermore, while interbody fusions are less likely to go on to reoperation,[12,13] one must weigh the risks of increased operation time, complications, and blood loss[10,13] before electing to undergo TLIF.

In recent years, improvements in technique and imaging have led to a trend toward more minimally invasive TLIF procedures (MIS). The traditional open technique requires a large soft tissue dissection to expose anatomic landmarks for pedicle screw fixation, leading to increased postoperative pain, longer recovery, and impaired spinal function.[2] In contrast, minimally invasive surgery allows for reduced surgical invasiveness with smaller wounds, limited blood loss, shorter hospital stays, and faster recovery.[2,14] MIS techniques often take longer to complete, which could be attributed to the learning curve needed to master the operations.[2] Advances in graft delivery arm systems have improved graft placement in the intervertebral space. Shau et al. demonstrated how an articulatory delivery arm system was able to place a graft in a 35% more anterior location, therefore allowing for increased segmental lordosis compared with traditional straight delivery arm systems.[15]

REFERENCES

1. Harms J, Rolinger H. A one-stager procedure in operative treatment of spondylolistheses: Dorsal traction-reposition and anterior fusion (author's transl). *Z Orthop Ihre Grenzgeb.* 1982; 120: 343–347.
2. Peng CW, Yue WM, Poh SY, Yeo W, Tan SB. Clinical and radiological outcomes of minimally invasive versus open transforaminal lumbar interbody fusion. *Spine.* 2009; 34(13): 1385–1389.
3. Jagannathan J, Sansur CA, Oskouian RJ, Fu KM, Shaffrey CI. Radiographic restoration of lumbar alignment after transforaminal lumbar interbody fusion. *Neurosurgery.* 2009; 64(5): 955–963.
4. Mummaneni PV, Rodts GE. The mini-open transforaminal lumbar interbody fusion. *Operative Neurosurgery.* 2005; 57(4): 256–261.
5. Chastain CA, Eck JC, Hodges SD, Humphreys SC, Levi P. Transforaminal lumbar interbody fusion: A retrospective study of long-term pain relief and fusion outcomes. *Orthopedics.* 2007; 30(5): 389–392.
6. Salehi SA, Tawk R, Ganju A, Lamarca F, Liu JC, Ondra SL. Transforaminal lumbar interbody fusion: Surgical technique and results in 24 patients. *Neurosurgery.* 2004; 54(2): 368–374.
7. Potter BK, Freedman BA, Verwiebe EG, Hall JM, Polly DW, Kuklo TR. Transforaminal lumbar interbody fusion: Clinical and radiographic results and complications in 100 consecutive patients. *J Spinal Disord Tech.* 2005; 18(4): 337–346.
8. Ahn DK, Park HS, Choi DJ, et al. The difference of surgical site infection according to the methods of lumbar fusion surgery. *J Spinal Disord Tech.* 2012; 25(8): E230–E234.
9. Audat Z, Moutasem O, Yousef K, Mohammad B. Comparison of clinical and radiological results of posterolateral fusion, posterior lumbar interbody fusion and transforaminal lumbar interbody fusion techniques in the treatment of degenerative lumbar spine. *Singapore Med J.* 2012; 53(3): 183–187.
10. Høy K, Bünger C, Niederman B, et al. Transforaminal lumbar interbody fusion (TLIF) versus posterolateral instrumented fusion (PLF) in degenerative lumbar disorders: A randomized clinical trial with 2-year follow-up. *Eur Spine J.* 2013; 22(9): 2022–2029.
11. Al Barbarawi MM, Audat ZM, Allouh MZ. Analytical comparison study of the clinical and radiological outcome of spine fixation using posterolateral, posterior lumber interbody and transforaminal lumber interbody spinal fixation techniques to treat lumber spine degenerative disc disease. *Scoliosis.* 2015; 10: 17.
12. Bydon M, Macki M, Abt NB, et al. The cost-effectiveness of interbody fusions versus posterolateral fusions in 137 patients with lumbar spondylolisthesis. *Spine J.* 2015; 15(3): 492–498.
13. Jalalpour K, Neumann P, Johansson C, Hedlund R. A randomized controlled trial comparing transforaminal lumbar interbody fusion and uninstrumented posterolateral fusion in the degenerative lumbar spine. *Global Spine J.* 2015; 5(4): 322–328.
14. Brodano GB, Martikos K, Lolli F, et al. Transforaminal lumbar interbody fusion in degenerative disk disease and spondylolisthesis Grade I: Minimally invasive versus open surgery. *J Spinal Disord Tech.* 2015; 28(10): E559–E564.
15. Shau DN, Parker SL, Mendenhall SK, et al. Transforaminal lumbar interbody graft placement using an articulating delivery arm facilitates increased segmental lordosis with superior anterior and midline graft placement. *J Spinal Disord Tech.* 2015; 28(4): 140–146.

CHAPTER 48

Spinal Cord Injury without Radiographic Abnormality in Children—The SCIWORA Syndrome

Pang D, Pollack IF. J Trauma 29(5):654–664, 1989

Reviewed by Daniel R. Kramer and Erin N. Kiehna

Research Question/Objective Spinal cord injuries in children are extremely rare; however, acute diagnosis in this population is challenging. The juvenile spine has inherent elasticity that allows for self-reduction of intersegmental injuries, which results in a normal appearing clinical radiograph. In 1982, the term *spinal cord injury without radiographic abnormality* (SCIWORA) was coined to explain the occurrence of spinal cord injury in the setting of normal plain radiographs and the absence of fracture on computed tomography (CT). This study reports a series of such cases to better describe the phenomenon and offer recommendations for management of SCIWORA.

Study Design A single institution retrospective chart review of a series of pediatric patients with evidence of traumatic myelopathy, without radiographic evidence of spinal injury (fracture or subluxation) on plain film X-ray, linear tomography, or computed tomography (CT).

Sample Size A total of 55 patients presenting to the pediatric level 1 trauma center at Children's Hospital of Pittsburgh between 1960 and 1989.

Follow-Up Biweekly through the period in which they wore a brace, then for 1 year past the injury.

Inclusion/Exclusion Criteria Inclusion criteria were not expressly listed; however, age range was 16 years old or younger. All patients received complete cervical spine films including open-mouth odontoid views. Exclusion criteria included patients with injury from birth trauma, penetrating injury, congenital abnormalities, or electric shock.

Intervention This was a retrospective review and thus the intervention was not being overtly examined; however, all patients were treated with the following minimum interventions: immediate resuscitation by a combined neurosurgical and trauma team. Rigid immobilization was employed as early as possible and throughout resuscitation. Complete spinal films were obtained as mentioned above.

Results   Patients were classified by injury location and type, dividing them into categories of upper cervical (C1-C4, $n = 10$), lower cervical (C5-C8, $n = 33$), upper thoracic (T1-T6, $n = 6$), and lower thoracic (T7-T12, $n = 6$). The majority of injuries were from motor vehicle accidents ($n = 28$), with falls the next most common ($n = 13$). The proposed mechanism of injury, inferred from witness testimony, involved flexion in the vast majority in the vast majority, with the next most common types of force including hyperextension and crush injury. Central cord was the most common type of injury to the cord ($n = 17$), followed by complete transection ($n = 12$), and mild partial cord injury ($n = 12$), with six instances of Brown-Séquard and four cases each of severe central and partial cord injury. Severe neurologic injury occurred most commonly with upper cervical and upper thoracic injuries. These severe upper cervical injuries were also most common with patients under 8 years old (after which the cervical spine takes on more adult-like characteristics). Dynamic flexion/extension plain films were performed to rule out overt instability. Patients with SCIWORA were immobilized in either a Philadelphia collar or a Guilford cervical brace for 8 to 12 weeks. Dynamic films were again obtained at the end of the bracing period. Somatosensory evoked potentials were obtained in 22 patients and were abnormal in 17, aiding in the differentiation of cranial and spinal cord injuries while also serving as a baseline to gauge recovery. The initial neurologic status provided the most reliable predictor of neurological outcome. Complete cord transection was either fatal or had no neurologic recovery. Severe cord injury recovery was related to level, with thoracic patients demonstrating improvement to independence. The mild to moderate cord injuries faired the best, with 26 children returning to a normal neurologic baseline. Delayed onset of neurologic deficits was seen in 27% of the patients. Deficits occurred an average of 1.4 days from injury (range, 30 minutes to 4 days). Nine of the patients had transient symptoms, with paresthesias in six, subjective weakness in three, and a "lightning" sensation down the spine in two. None of the patients with delayed symptoms were initially immobilized. Two of these patients progressed to complete transection and four to severe cord injury. Another eight patients displayed a second spinal cord injury 3 days to 10 weeks after the initial injury (delayed SCIWORA), which, in all cases, was a mild partial cervical cord injury. Despite prior immobilization, only two of eight patients were wearing their collar/brace. Repeat imaging, including dynamic plain films and one magnetic resonance imaging (MRI) study, were normal. For the eight patients with a second SCIWORA, four children had permanent disability.

This study demonstrates that the unique laxity of the pediatric spine allows for spinal column deformation resulting in spinal cord injury without showing plain film or CT evidence of instability. The authors offer their recommendations: stringent immobilization with a Guilford brace, an orthotic brace not easily removed and with anterior and posterior support, for three months. Strict limits on sports, including noncontact sports, are maintained. Dynamic films are completed after the 3 months of immobilization.

Study Limitations   This was a retrospective review over a substantial period of time (1960–1987). Diagnostic and treatment protocols changed vastly over this time, even though this is a single institutional study. Radiographs were the standard diagnostic film, with CT being obtained only afterward. Based on mechanism of injury alone, the majority of these patients would receive a CT scan as part of their trauma workup in the modern era. MRI was only available at the end of their study, and indeed only one patient underwent MRI. The very concept of SCIWORA is without MRI and thus lacks the diagnostic potential of modern-day management. MRI can demonstrate fractures through the disc spaces and ligamentous instability/rupture that would not necessarily be visible on CT or radiographs. MRI can also show bony edema representative of growth plate distraction in children. Although the series is large for such a rare entity, the numbers themselves are limited, with merely 12 thoracic injuries, severely reducing generalizability. Similarly, although the delayed deficit is alarming, the rarity makes any conclusions difficult to interpret. Additionally, the management recommendations are not validated.

Relevant Studies   SCIWORA is an extremely important concept in pediatric trauma, and Pang and Pollack identify and characterize the phenomenon in children under 16 years old. Since that time, their findings have been echoed in a number of reviews, most notably a series of 174 cases, where again, patients under 10 years old were more likely to have high cervical injuries and more severe spinal cord injuries.[1] An updated review by Pang in 2004 solidifies the ideas purported in their original 1989 study, including the at-risk demographic and mechanisms of injury. Biomechanical studies, summarized in his review, help confirm the underlying pathophysiology among young children: The ligaments are more elastic; the facets have a more horizontal orientation; high water content in the disc allows for easier mobilization; the segments slip more readily due to anterior positions; the uncinate processes are unformed, allowing lateral movement; the growth zone is susceptible to fracture; and the head is disproportionally heavy compared to neck strength. Most of these issues are resolved as the pediatric neck becomes a more adult-like spine around 9 years old, reflecting the increased incidence of high cervical and severe injuries in those less than 9 years old.[3]

This study was conducted prior to the use of MRI. Since that time, MRI has become an important addition to the management of these patients. Patients with SCIWORA evaluated with MRI exhibited abnormal MRI findings in 22%–65%, and those with abnormal findings were more likely to have persistent

neurologic deficits at discharge.[2,3] Recent studies have made updated recommendations that include the addition of an MRI, complete plain films or CT scan of
the entire spine, as well as immediate and posttreatment flexion/extension films
after treatment with immobilization. They also loosen recommendations for
length of immobilization on those that are asymptomatic and have confirmed
stability on dynamic films, but they extend abstinence from high-risk activities
through 6 months.[3,4]

REFERENCES

1. Hamilton MG, Myles ST. Pediatric spinal injury: Review of 174 hospital admissions.
   J Neurosurg. 1992; 77: 700–704.
2. Mahajan P, Jaffe DM, Olsen CS, et al. Spinal cord injury without radiologic abnormality in
   children imaged with magnetic resonance imaging. *J Trauma Acute Care Surg.* 2013; 75:
   843–847.
3. Pang D. Spinal cord injury without radiographic abnormality in children, 2 decades later.
   Neurosurgery. 2004; 55: 1325–1342; discussion 1342–1323.
4. Rozzelle CJ, Aarabi B, Dhall SS, et al. Spinal cord injury without radiographic abnormality
   (SCIWORA). *Neurosurgery.* 2013; 72(Suppl2): 227–233.

CHAPTER 49

Pediatric Spinal Trauma: Review of 122 Cases of Spinal Cord and Vertebral Column Injuries*

Hadley MN, Zabramski JM, Browner CM, et al. J Neurosurgery 68(1):18–24, 1988

Reviewed by Jetan H. Badhiwala and Peter B. Dirks

Research Question/Objective Pediatric spinal injuries are uncommon. The developing pediatric spine has several anatomical and biomechanical features that distinguish it from the mature adult spine and, accordingly, one would expect a distinct injury profile in children. In a time when there was very limited clinical data on pediatric spine trauma, Hadley and colleagues sought to evaluate injury patterns, treatment options, and clinical outcomes of spinal trauma in children and moreover the relationship, if any, of age with etiology of injury, injury type, spinal level of injury, and incidence and degree of associated neurological compromise.

Study Design This was a retrospective case series of children treated at the Barrow Neurological Institute from July 1972 to July 1986. Patients were divided into three categories based on age (0 to 9 years, 10 to 14 years, or 15 to 16 years) to facilitate comparison of mechanism of injury, injury pattern and level, and incidence and degree of neurological compromise with age. Neurological function was graded according to the Frankel classification system.[1] Chi-square tests were used to analyze differences among age groups.

Sample Size There were 122 patients included ($n = 122$).

Follow-Up Follow-up data was available for 113 of 122 patients (93%), with a median follow-up period of 44 months (range, 1 month to 10 years).

Inclusion/Exclusion Criteria Pediatric patients (<16 years) with acute vertebral column or spinal cord injuries were eligible. Patients

---

* Hadley MN, Zabramski JM, Browner CM, Rekate H, Sonntag VK. Pediatric spinal trauma: Review of 122 cases of spinal cord and vertebral column injuries. *J Neurosurg.* 1988; 68(1): 18–24.

with penetrating injuries to the spine or those with injuries associated with congenital vertebral column anomalies were excluded.

Intervention or Treatment Received   Surgical stabilization or nonoperative treatment, including bedrest or one of several forms of external immobilization.

Results   The most common mechanisms of injury were motor vehicle collision (MVC; 39%), fall (15%), sports injury (11%), and pedestrian-automobile accident (11%). Falls and pedestrian-automobile accidents caused the majority of injuries among the 0- to 9-year-old age group, whereas 15- and 16-year-olds were most frequently injured in MVCs. There were four distinct injury patterns: fracture only (41%), fracture with subluxation (33%), subluxation only (10%), and spinal cord injury without radiographic abnormality (SCIWORA; 16%). There was a higher incidence of subluxation-only injuries and SCIWORA among children 0 to 9 years of age. On the other hand, 10- to 16-year-olds mostly sustained fracture or fracture/subluxation injuries. The presence of subluxation conferred higher risk of neurological injury. At admission, 50% of patients were neurologically intact, and 33% had incomplete and 17% complete spinal cord injuries. The incidence of neurological injury was higher among the 0- to 9-year-old group. The majority of injuries in 0- to 9-year-olds involved the cervical spine (72%), most commonly between the occiput and C2. The levels of injuries among the 15- and 16-year age group was similar to the distribution of spinal injuries in the adult population. The rate of multi-level injury was 16%. Most patients (84%) were managed nonoperatively, ranging from bedrest and a foam collar to external immobilization with a halo vest or bivalve body jacket. Sixteen percent of patients underwent surgery as primary treatment for fracture, fracture/subluxation, or subluxation only. An additional three patients required delayed surgery for failure of nonoperative treatment. No patient in the cohort deteriorated as a result of therapy. Of the 38 patients with incomplete spinal cord injuries at admission available for follow-up, eight improved two Frankel grades, 26 improved one Frankel grade, and four patients were unchanged. Of the 20 patients available for follow-up review who had complete spinal cord injuries, three died, three improved three Frankel grades to Grade D, one improved to Grade C, and 13 had no improvement (Grade A). Of the patients with SCIWORA, those in the 0- to 9-year age group had greater neurological compromise and poorer recovery.

Study Limitations   This study is limited primarily by a retrospective design, which by nature is prone to missing and inaccurate data. Despite being one of the larger series of pediatric spinal injuries, the sample size is still relatively small. Many of the statistical comparisons did not reach significance, and we suspect this is primarily a power issue. The authors do not comment on the incidence and severity of concomitant injuries, including head injuries, which can be an important source of morbidity and mortality in the pediatric trauma population. This data would be useful considering these patients often have multisystem injuries, and their care requires an interdisciplinary team of health care professionals.

Relevant Studies Many early studies provided insight into the biomechanics of the developing spine. These suggested that the pediatric spine is relatively hypermobile due to several distinct anatomical features (including ligamentous laxity; underdevelopment of the neck and paraspinal musculature; absent uncinate processes; incompletely ossified wedge-shaped vertebrae; and shallow, horizontally oriented facets) explaining the phenomenon of pseudosubluxation.[1–7] Yet there remained little clinical data on spinal trauma in children. The present paper was one of the earliest and largest case series of pediatric spinal injuries to be published in the literature, and its findings provided much needed insight into the clinical implications of the biomechanical features of the immature spine in the setting of trauma. Several important conclusions can be drawn from the work of Hadley and colleagues, and these remain relevant in the modern era. First, young children are less prone to fracture and more prone to subluxation. The elasticity of the pediatric spine appears to be protective against relatively minor trauma that may otherwise result in fracture in the more mature, rigid spine; however, the same hypermobility makes young children more prone to subluxation injuries, SCIWORA, and more severe neurological injury after trauma involving relatively greater force. Second, young children are especially susceptible to cervical spine injuries, in particular between the occiput and C2. In a series of 71 children, Ruge et al. found this to be especially true for children 3 years of age or younger.[8] This is explained by the large size of the head relative to the torso, which shifts the fulcrum of movement to the upper cervical spine, with flexion and extension centered at C2-C3. On the other hand, adolescents with a more mature, adult-like spine have similar injury types and patterns to those observed in adult patients. Furthermore, operative stabilization is infrequently required, and the outcome after pediatric spinal trauma is generally favorable.

Some of the limitations of the present work were overcome by subsequent studies. Hamilton and Myles published their experience with 174 children with spinal injuries at the University of Calgary in 1992.[9] Their findings essentially mirrored those of Hadley et al., but the larger sample size resulted in several statistical comparisons being significant, whereas many of these were only trends in the earlier paper. In particular, the higher incidence of SCIWORA, occiput to C2 injuries, neurological injury, and injuries secondary to falls and pedestrian-automobile accidents among 0- to 9-year-olds compared to older age groups all reached statistical significance. In 2004, Carreon and associates reviewed 137 hospital admissions for pediatric spine fractures.[10] Unlike Hadley et al., the authors of this work also examined associated injuries, which were seen in 53% of the cohort and included head injuries (26%), extraspinal fractures (21%), abdominal injuries (16%), and pneumothoraces/hemothoraces (12%). Head injuries were commonly associated with cervical spine injuries.

The incidence of SCIWORA has been a topic of debate in the literature. Pang and Wilberger first described SCIWORA in 1982 in a series of children with objective signs of traumatic myelopathy with no radiographic evidence of fracture or subluxation.[11] SCIWORA is thought to result from the mismatch in the elasticity of the vertebral column and spinal cord. Leventhal's 1960 cadaveric study found the neonatal spinal column could be stretched 2 inches without structural disruption, whereas the spinal cord ruptures after only ¼ inch of stretching.[12] Hadley et al. found the incidence of SCIWORA among children with spinal cord injury to be 33%. This is in contrast to the 67% frequency reported in Pang and Wilberger's original series, but it is similar to the 35% reported by Osenbach and Menezes and the 28% reported by Hamilton and Myles.[9,11,13] In a review of the literature, Pang found a mean incidence of 34.8% for SCIWORA among children 17 years or younger with spinal cord injury.[14]

REFERENCES

1. Frankel HL, Hancock DO, Hyslop G, et al. The value of postural reduction in the initial management of closed injuries of the spine with paraplegia and tetraplegia. I. *Paraplegia.* 1969; 7(3): 179–192.
2. Fesmire FM, Luten RC. The pediatric cervical spine: Developmental anatomy and clinical aspects. *J Emerg Med.* 1989; 7(2): 133–142.
3. Townsend EH Jr., Rowe ML. Mobility of the upper cervical spine in health and disease. *Pediatrics.* 1952; 10(5): 567–574.
4. Papavasiliou V. Traumatic subluxation of the cervical spine during childhood. *Orthop Clin North Am.* 1978; 9(4): 945–954.
5. Sherk HH, Schut L, Lane JM. Fractures and dislocations of the cervical spine in children. *Orthop Clin North Am.* 1976; 7(3): 593–604.
6. Cattell HS, Filtzer DL. Pseudosubluxation and other normal variations in the cervical spine in children: A study of one hundred and sixty children. *J Bone Joint Surg Am.* 1965; 47(7): 1295–1309.
7. Bailey DK. The normal cervical spine in infants and children. *Radiology.* 1952; 59(5): 712–719.
8. Ruge JR, Sinson GP, McLone DG, Cerullo LJ. Pediatric spinal injury: The very young. *J Neurosurg.* 1988; 68(1): 25–30.
9. Hamilton MG, Myles ST. Pediatric spinal injury: Review of 174 hospital admissions. *J Neurosurg.* 1992; 77(5): 700–704.
10. Carreon LY, Glassman SD, Campbell MJ. Pediatric spine fractures: A review of 137 hospital admissions. *J Spinal Disord Tech.* 2004; 17(6): 477–482.
11. Pang D, Wilberger JE Jr. Spinal cord injury without radiographic abnormalities in children. *J Neurosurg.* 1982; 57(1): 114–129.
12. Leventhal HR. Birth injuries of the spinal cord. *J Pediatr.* 1960; 56: 447–453.
13. Osenbach RK, Menezes AH. Spinal cord injury without radiographic abnormality in children. *Pediatr Neurosci.* 1989; 15(4): 168–174; discussion 175.
14. Pang D. Spinal cord injury without radiographic abnormality in children, 2 decades later. *Neurosurgery.* 2004; 55(6): 1325–1342; discussion 1342–1323.

CHAPTER 50

The Tethered Spinal Cord: Its Protean Manifestations, Diagnosis, and Surgical Correction

Hoffman HJ, Hendrick EB, Humphreys RP. Child's Brain 2(3):145–155, 1976

Reviewed by Arjun V. Pendharkar, Raphael Guzman, and Samuel H. Cheshier

Research Question/Objective The clinical entity of tethered cord has evolved significantly over the past 100 years. Several early reports had described a progressive neurological deficit in the context of a fixed spinal cord, but varying theories implicated thickened filum terminale, lipoma, myelomeningocele, and other associated pathologies. The present study aimed to further characterize the tethered cord syndrome in the absence of other obvious spinal dysraphisms and describe the clinical outcomes after laminectomy and surgical sectioning of the filum terminale.

Study Design A clinical review was conducted of children who underwent surgical release of a tethered spinal cord.

Sample Size Thirty-one children treated at the Hospital for Sick Children in Toronto, Canada, were included in this study.

Follow-Up Duration of follow-up was not outlined in the manuscript.

Inclusion/Exclusion Criteria All 31 patients presented with back pain, scoliosis, progressive lower extremity weakness, or neurogenic bladder, and had lumbosacral spina bifida occulta. Supine myelography with pantopague demonstrated a low position of the conus medullaris (below L2). Several of the patients also had a thickened filum (2 mm or greater in diameter). Excluded were those patients with lipomyelomeningoceles; meningoceles; myelomeningoceles; diastematomyelia; or intraspinal space-occupying dysraphic conditions, including dermoid tumors, intraspinal meningoceles, neurenteric cysts, and teratomatous cysts.

Intervention   Patients underwent a lumbosacral laminectomy and surgical release of the tethered spinal cord. Upward movement of the proximal filum or spinal cord ranged from 1 cm to 2.5 cm. Two patients with scoliosis further underwent Harrington fusion.

Results   Intraoperatively, 19 patients had a thickened fibrotic filum terminale. One patient had a intrafilar cyst, and seven patients had instrinsic lipomas within the filum. Four patients had no filum and instead had a small lipomatous connection at the end of the dural sac. There was upward movement of the cord or proximal filum (ranging from 1–2.5 cm) in all patients. Of the 26 patients who presented with motor/sensory loss, 23 did not need their future planned orthopedic corrective procedure. There were six children with bowel and/or bladder incontinence and all experienced improvement or return to normal function. All seven patients who presented with pain had complete resolution of their symptoms.

Study Limitations   In this study, the time course of clinical follow-up is not reported, and thus it remains unclear whether there was an acute improvement in function after tethered cord release and how durable the results were in the long term. The authors describe the tethered cord syndrome but exclude many common causes of tethered cord, including lipoma, myelomeningocele, and other dysraphic malformations. The syndrome may have been better termed *simple tethered cord*. It is interesting that the authors found three fat pads concurrent with a thickened tethered filum terminale without any associated large lipoma. Another limitation is the clinical endpoints used. For example, there are no urodynamic data but rather the subjective assessment of a urologist in evaluating bowel and bladder function. Furthermore, improvements in motor function, sensory function, reflexes, and degree of scoliosis were not presented in any objective manner, only to note that "improvements" were seen. Nonetheless, given the limitations in imaging available at the time, this paper is remarkable in describing good surgical outcomes after untethering of the filum terminale and remains a landmark study in pediatric neurosurgery.

Relevant Studies   This study laid the groundwork for future progress in the diagnosis and management of simple tethered cord. For example, the pathophysiology of tethered cord has been studied extensively and is thought to be due to stretch-induced impairments in oxidative metabolism. When in conjunction with dysraphic conditions like lipomyelomeningocele, there may also be local mass effect on the cord. As introduced in this study, urodynamic testing is a critical portion of the workup for tethered cord. More recent studies have validated urodynamic studies in predicting future neurosurgical intervention. Expanding on the findings from the primary paper, surgeons have gone on to release tethered cords associated with many different pathological entities and variations of spinal dysraphisms, with good clinical outcomes. There remains considerable debate, however, on timing of intervention and the role of early/prophylactic untethering in the asymptomatic patient with radiographic tethered cord.

BIBLIOGRAPHY

1. Fuchs A. Über Beziehungen der Enuresis Nocturna zu Rudimentarformen der Spina Bifida Occulta (Myelodysplasie). *Wien Med Wochenschr*. 1910; 80: 1569–1573.
2. Yamada S, Zinke DE, Sanders D. Pathophysiology of "tethered cord syndrome." *J Neurosurg*. 1981; 54: 494–503.
3. Yamada S, Won DJ, Perzeshkpour G, et al. Pathophysiology of tethered cord syndrome and similar disorders. *Neurosurg Focus*. 2007; 23: 2E6.
4. Lavallée LT, Leonard MP, Dubois C, Guerra LA. Urodynamic testing—is it a useful tool in the management of children with cutaneous stigmata of occult spinal dysraphism? *J Urol*. 2013; 189(2): 678–683.
5. Guerra LA, Pike J, Milks J, Barrowman N, Leonard M. Outcome in patients who underwent tethered cord release for occult spinal dysraphism. *J Urol*. 2006; 176(4 Pt 2): 1729–1732.
6. White JT, Samples DC, Prieto JC, Tarasiewicz I. Systematic review of urologic outcomes from tethered cord release in occult spinal dysraphism in children. *Curr Urol Rep*. 2015; 16(11): 1–13, http://doi.org/10.1007/s11934-015-0550-6.

Index

Note: Page numbers followed by f and t refer to figures and tables, respectively.

Printed in the United States
by Baker & Taylor Publisher Services